THE

PARADOX

OF FINE

A Midlife Health
Transformation

by

MATT BRAND

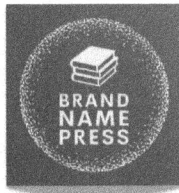

The Paradox of Fine: A Midlife Health Transformation
Publisher: Matt Brand

ISBN: 979-8-9922854-0-6
e-ISBN: 979-8-9922854-1-3

First Edition
Printed in the USA

ABOUT THE AUTHOR

A self-proclaimed (and peer-verified) nerd, Matt Brand balances life as a father of two teenage daughters, software engineer, local school board member, and advocate for better-than-fine living. He believes he is quite funny. His daughters disagree. They believe he is "mostly cringe." His deep roots in summer camp culture and his journey through parenthood inspired his debut book, "Nature & Nurture: A Journey Through the Fog of Parenting" (2024). His ridiculously high cholesterol inspired "The Paradox of Fine: A Midlife Health Transformation." When not writing, working, or perfecting dad jokes, he can be found in his home gym near Boston, where his daughters continue to decline his invitations to work out together.

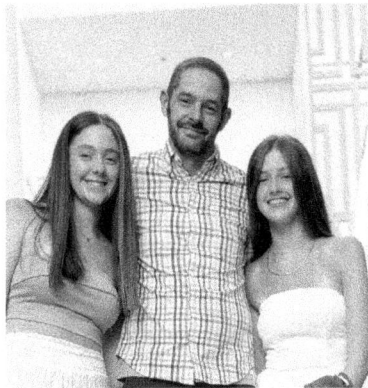

To Julianna, Chloe, and my entire family:
Thank you for tolerating my wacky ideas and accepting my awkwardness. Thanks for accepting my shenanigans.

To Danyael:
This journey would not have been successful without your support, patience, food ideas, and general help every step of the way. I know it's not always easy to be around someone who won't stop doing things and I appreciate that you respect me for being me. Love you.

Table of Contents

Part Three
Physical Evidence

Part Four
Unexpected Discoveries

Part Five
The Long View

INTRODUCTION

"The definition of insanity is doing something over and over again and expecting different results."

Albert Einstein

If only Einstein's definition of insanity were true for me as I got older — instead, my version might be "doing something over and over again and expecting the same results." When I started writing my first book, "Nature & Nurture: A Journey Through the Fog of Parenting," I figured I'd be one and done. The idea of writing — and ultimately publishing — a book was quite daunting. I have spent the bulk of my professional career as a software engineer at startup companies. While I have always enjoyed writing, I never considered myself to be a writer. That being said, when I was around 75% of the way through writing that book, my overactive brain started forming seeds of other ideas I'd had.

During this time, I was also well into a significant set of changes to the way I was living my life in an attempt to get healthier. Before starting my first book, I struggled with trying to reconcile why anyone would read a book that I wrote. While I'm a parent, I'm not an expert. I had a goal to try and write in a way that was centered around my own experience as a parent but would hopefully not be preachy or prescriptive. My hope was that someone would read it and reflect on their own experiences as a parent. As I made my way through that book, I started feeling better and better about achieving that goal the further I got.

One of the ideas was to write about the health and fitness journey I was on. I wondered if I could use a similar tone and style and center the narrative around my own experience but write it in a way that I hoped would be informative enough and approachable enough that others could read it and hopefully find it similarly relatable. That seed started to grow into a sapling and ultimately became "The Paradox of Fine: A Midlife Health Transformation."

This is a book about my health transformation that really started during the summer of 2021, when I was about to turn 43 years old. A routine annual doctor's appointment revealed dangerously bad cholesterol levels that surprised me — although really shouldn't have had I paid better attention to my health as I got older and in particular as I entered my forties. After years of making poor health choices that did not seem to affect me in any way I could discern — other than what I wrote off as normal physical changes to my body that "everyone" experiences as they get older — I just assumed that I was fine. It enabled me to get comfortable and complacent. This is the paradox. I was living "fine" which was masking my ability to actually be fine, or better.

Being 'fine' is both a comfort and a trap. We all do it — accept little compromises, write off changes as 'just getting older,' tell ourselves that good enough is, well, good enough. Maybe it's that extra flight of stairs that now leaves us winded, or those jeans that mysteriously shrunk in the wash, or that energy we used to have but can't quite find anymore. We label these changes as normal, expected, fine. But what if 'fine' is just another word for settling? What if it's keeping us from discovering what lies beyond it?

After that fateful doctor's appointment, I learned very quickly that I had a lot to learn; and not just about cholesterol.

This book and the journey within from 'fine' to something better unfolds across five parts. We'll start where I did — in the comfort of 'fine,' where a routine doctor's visit shattered my illusions about health. Then we'll dive into the crucial moment of choosing change, when knowing you need to do something becomes actually doing it. As the story progresses, we'll explore not just the physical evidence of transformation, but also the unexpected discoveries that emerge when you start questioning one aspect of your life and end up questioning everything. Finally, we'll look at the long view — because real change isn't about quick fixes or temporary solutions, it's about building a sustainable future that's decidedly better.

My hope for you isn't that after you read it you will know the exact set of steps that are necessary for you to take in order to achieve whatever your goals are. That wouldn't be possible for a few reasons: I am not a personal trainer. I'm not an expert in exercise science. I am not a nutritionist. I am not you.

In my business life — and in building software in particular — I frequently find myself asking "why?" In doing so I am trying to get to the core problem that we, as a team, are trying to solve. That is where my health journey started as well. If you don't know what you're solving for then it is not likely you'll solve it. Once you do know (and maybe you do already), you can figure out your plan of attack.

Getting older isn't an excuse to be complacent. Getting older does not have to be a reason to just accept that what your life is today is what your life has to be tomorrow. While change is often hard for many people — and it gets harder and more challenging as we age — it is never too late to make one. Once you commit to a change you might end up in a similar situation as mine. You might end up learning things about yourself that you were totally unaware of that are actually far bigger and more impactful than cholesterol.

You'll never know until you try…

Actually, as my good friend Yoda once said, "No. Try not. Do… or do not. There is no try."

Be Yoda. He was 900 years old when he died and lived a very eventful life.

Do.

PART ONE

THE COMFORT OF FINE

CHAPTER ONE

NUMBERS DON'T LIE

1

For 40 years, I thought being thin meant being healthy. It was a simple equation: if you could see your toes when you looked down, you were probably fine. My annual physicals reinforced this belief — normal blood pressure, steady weight, decent BMI. I had mastered the art of being 'fine.'

July 20, 2021, 7:00 am, changed all that.

I arrived at the doctor's office that morning the same way I had for years: confident, unbothered, and maybe even a little smug about my supposedly good health...

I checked in and waited to be called. After a few minutes (I was one of the first appointments of the day), I heard my name and followed a nurse to the exam room. Per the normal routine, I stepped on the scale for my weight. 166 pounds (plus 6.4 ounces). She took my temperature and blood pressure. At a temperature of 97.9 degrees Fahrenheit and a blood pressure reading of 116/70, everything was, once again, looking good. I am 6'1" tall so my Body Mass Index[1] (BMI) was 21.95. A good BMI for a man in his 40s like I was, about to turn 44 at the time, is anywhere between 19.0 and 26.9. My score was almost right in the middle of the acceptable range.

My vitals were all good. This was a general pattern I had grown accustomed to over the previous 40-plus years.

The nurse finished her checks and told me to sit tight; Kaitie would be in soon. Kaitie is a nurse practitioner and has been my primary care physician for many years. I originally had a doctor as my PCP but prior to my first appointment, I got a call that he was not able to see me. I was given the choice to reschedule or meet with one of the nurse practitioners. I opted for the latter. After all, I had a long history of nothing-burgers at these appointments so I might as well just keep the schedule and get on with it. This is when I first met Kaitie.

It happened again the next year and I met with Kaitie a second time. After that visit, I just started scheduling with her. It was easier and I like consistency. Now, for all intents and purposes, Kaitie was my doctor and I was thrilled. I look for consistency in providers like this. I don't want to be starting from zero every time I have an appointment and I want to work with people who don't sugarcoat things. I can make my own decisions but please just tell me how it is.

---

[1] According to the Centers for Disease Control (CDC), Body Mass Index (BMI) is a measure of weight relative to height. It is just one metric but is a quick and easy way to determine if someone is underweight, overweight, obese, or within the normal range. It is calculated by taking a person's weight in kilograms and dividing it by the square of their height in meters.

Anyhow, a few minutes after the nurse left the room, Kaitie came in. We chatted as we normally do about how the year had gone, if there had been any major life changes, how my kids were, how I was feeling, and so on. Once we finished that part of the check-in, she conducted the standard exam. How was my vision? Fine. How about those reflexes? Fine. Say "Ahhhh." Fine. She did all the standard things and once again, everything looked normal. I usually think to myself, "It must be quite boring to have me as a patient."

For all these years, nothing ever changes. I've always been relatively healthy. I've never been overweight. Another good exam with Kaitie in the books. See you next year.

Kaitie lets me know that the nurse will be back in to get my blood. I wouldn't say I'm a huge fan of needles to the point of looking forward to a blood draw but I'm a trooper and can manage just fine. Once Kaitie heads out the nurse comes right back in as if she had been waiting right outside the door. She looks at my arms to determine which she will target and her eyes light up. This is also a common occurrence with me. I have A-plus vein visibility. I never thought that the veins in my arms would make anyone so happy but am happy to bring so much joy to this nurse and so many others over the years.

She takes the requisite blood and gives me the boring bandaid. How I long for the days of Smurf bandaids. Most of the time it takes until the end of the day, at least, for the bloodwork to come in and for Kaitie to have the time to look at it and send me the notes. I headed home because I was working from home that day.

I got home and had a normal and largely forgettable day of work.

Later in the afternoon, my cell phone rang. It was Kaitie. Normally she wouldn't call. Normally, she would just add some visit notes to my medical record that I could access through an app on my phone. When I answered she didn't seem panicked or anything so I was curious as to why she was calling. She told me she had reviewed my bloodwork and wanted to discuss some things with me.

Uh oh.

Much of my bloodwork was clinically normal and good. But my cholesterol? How do I say this with the proper gravity? It was not good. Kaitie proceeded to tell me the various scores for my cholesterol. It's worth noting that at this point in my life, I had a very limited understanding of what I thought cholesterol was. Essentially, my understanding at the time was that cholesterol, in general, is bad. My understanding was that it was some sort of "gunk" that would clog up your arteries and it would build up from various types of food (like fast food). That was about all I knew.

So here's Kaitie telling me that my triglycerides were at 1036. The optimal number is under 150. My total cholesterol was 247 with an optimal range between 140 and 200. My HDL score was 36 and apparently, that's the good cholesterol and should be over 40. My cardiac risk factor was 6.9 and that should be below 5. I really had very little knowledge of what all this meant but I do understand numbers and know that all of those scores were outside the optimal range and the triglyceride number was WAY out of the optimal range.

July 2021 Bloodwork Results

Measure	Result	Optimal Range
Total Cholesterol	247	140-200
Calculated LDL	4	0-129, <100 optimal
Cardiac Risk	6.9	0-5
Triglycerides	1036	<150 optimal
HDL	36	>40 optimal
Non-HDL	211	---

My cholesterol was never considered to be wonderful but also was never concerning. Now, it was concerning; enough that Kaitie wanted to call me to discuss strategies for how we would move forward.

2

November, 2024

This is not a medical journal. I am not a doctor, scientist, or expert in health in any way. I am a 47-year-old man and I have spent the majority of my life thinking I was fine. Because of my fast metabolism, I could always eat anything I wanted. On most Sundays when I was in my twenties, I would wake up shortly after noon, drive to McDonald's, get a double quarter pounder with cheese, a large order of French fries, and an even larger Coca-Cola. I would get home, pop myself down on the couch, and spend the afternoon watching football. During this time, I suspect most people, including me, would see me and think that I was totally healthy. I was not overweight and while certainly not muscular looking, I, like most people who knew me, probably thought I was fine in terms of health.

For as long as I can remember, prior to July of 2021, I never worried about my health. If I looked fine I probably was. If it looks like chicken and tastes like chicken, it's probably chicken. For me, everything felt and seemed great right up until the moment it wasn't.

There are plenty of great resources for learning about cholesterol so this book will not be a comprehensive explanation of how it all works. I do however want to include my new understanding of the various types of cholesterol including how you acquire each type and how they affect your body. If you want an even greater discussion about cholesterol, I highly recommend you read a book written by Peter Attia, who is a doctor, called "Outlive: The Science & Art of Longevity." The 7th chapter of the book is all about cholesterol and gives a ton of great scientific information about the different types. It's an outstanding book in general filled with lots of great science and information about health and I highly recommend it.

That being said, I'm a software engineer and love a good research project. I needed to understand as best as I could to understand the basics about different types of cholesterol and related concepts:

First, according to heart.org[2], there are a number of misconceptions about people with high cholesterol:

- Thin people don't have high cholesterol. While it is more likely to have high cholesterol if you're overweight, being this does not make you immune to it.

- Men are the only people who need to worry about it. Not true.

- If you have high cholesterol, medications alone can solve your problem. Not true. The medication can certainly help but lifestyle changes are called for if you want to see sustained improvement.

HDL (High-Density Lipoprotein) - "The Good Cholesterol"

This cholesterol is good because it essentially acts as a housecleaner for your other cholesterol; the cholesterol that is less good for you. It essentially delivers the bad cholesterol to your liver for disposal. The higher the number the better.

LDL (Low-Density Lipoprotein) - "The Bad Cholesterol"

This is the stuff that builds up in your arteries and clogs the pipes. It is not good. You want this number to be low.

Triglycerides

---

[2] Common misconceptions about cholesterol:
https://www.heart.org/en/health-topics/cholesterol/about-cholesterol/common-misconceptions-about-cholesterol

Your body tries to burn calories for energy. Triglycerides are unused calories that get converted to fat and are stored in your body for later use. You want this number to be low. A number of things can cause an increase in triglycerides. Soda, sweets, and white bread are examples of foods that your body converts to triglycerides for storage. Fast foods, especially when you're eating a lot of carbohydrates and fats together would increase your triglycerides. Alcohol consumption can do it. Lack of exercise, high-stress levels, and not sleeping well are all contributors.

Cardiac Risk Ratio

This is calculated by dividing your total cholesterol by your HDL score. It is essentially a basic score that tells you the risk of heart disease. Of course, with your cardiac risk ratio, the lower the number the better. The total cholesterol is a combination of your HDL, LDL, and Triglycerides.

Visceral Fat

This is hidden fat that lives around your organs, mostly in your abdominal region. Too much of this can squeeze your organs and make it harder for them to do their job. It also actively produces hormones that can cause inflammation. Visceral fat is NOT the fat that you can pinch right under your skin. That kind of fat is called...

Subcutaneous Fat

This is the fat you can pinch (well, definitely not me - but probably you). This is more like a blanket around your body. It's actually considered to be less dangerous than visceral fat because it doesn't produce any hormones and it doesn't really get in the way of your organs. It is mostly used for energy storage.

Insulin

When you eat food, particularly food high in carbohydrates, or junk food, your blood sugar levels go up. This, as its name implies is the amount of sugar in your bloodstream. Your pancreas produces insulin. The insulin helps move sugar from your blood into your cells and your blood sugar levels go down. Once in the cells, there are a few options for that sugar. Some of it is broken down immediately into something called ATP, which stands for Adenosine Triphosphate, but let's be honest, I can't pronounce that so we'll stick with ATP. This is the energy your cells use to make your brain and muscles work. The other option for sugar in your cells is for it to get stored. It can be stored in your muscles and liver as something called glycogen or in fat cells as...fat. With glycogen, your body will convert it back into sugar when it detects low blood sugar and with the fat storage, your body can convert that into usable energy when it's needed.

Now let's talk about how they are all connected.

The worst-case scenario would be having high Triglycerides (like 1036) and low HDL (36) — which is exactly what I was dealing with. Okay, so why are these things so bad? We know that the triglycerides get converted to fat and stored for later use. What happens when you have too much of it and not enough places to put it in your body? It starts to accumulate in your body's tissue including around your organs. This directly contributes to the accumulation of visceral fat.

Because HDL's job is to clean up the bad cholesterol, when you don't have enough of it, your body isn't doing enough cleaning and the garbage continues to accumulate. We know that visceral fat produces hormones that cause inflammation. That inflammation causes insulin resistance. This creates more triglycerides and the spiral continues because you already don't have enough HDL to "fight back."

Insulin resistance is when your cells are no longer responding to the insulin as efficiently and not moving the sugar into your cells. This means that people with insulin resistance typically have higher blood sugar. It also does not mean that your pancreas stops producing insulin. It continues to do that. Now you have a lot of insulin and a lot of sugar in your blood. This set of events can eventually lead to Type 2 Diabetes.

The visceral fat that's forming around your organs and producing the hormones that cause inflammation is causing other problems too. That inflammation is damaging blood vessel walls which makes it easier for cholesterol to build up on those damaged walls. This build-up makes it so the vessels themselves are less flexible. This, naturally, means your heart has to work harder to pump blood through the less flexible vessels. Now your blood pressure goes up because everything is less efficient. Don't forget that the visceral fat can accumulate around your heart making it harder for the heart itself to pump. Because your blood flow is not as good as it should be, the risk of a blood clot goes up. There is also now an increase in plaque build-up in those vessels making them even narrower. These pieces of plaque can break off and form clots.

Think of it this way: maybe your blood vessels are a five-lane highway when they're healthy. Some giant flatbed truck dumps a bunch of cargo on a few of the lanes on one side, at rush hour. Now, all that traffic has to get where it's going in fewer lanes.

You might have already guessed where we're going. Any one of those things, from a piece of plaque breaking off and forming a clot to a vessel getting so narrow that nothing can get through, can cause a heart attack.

High triglycerides, low HDL, visceral fat, and inflammation are things that could contribute to an issue with your heart and they are all related.

While I'm still not a doctor, I feel like I know a lot more now than I did in July of 2021 about this stuff. The only question was...

3

July 20, 2021, late afternoon

...what am I going to do now?

Kaitie and I talked for a bit about some of the things I could try to deal with this problem. For the longest time, I felt and looked fine even as its definition changed as I got older. Now I was presented with an objective reality that I was not, in fact, fine. For the first time in my life, I couldn't just coast on being naturally thin. The numbers on my bloodwork didn't care about how my clothes fit or what I saw in the mirror — they were telling a different story entirely.

There were a few strategies that we went over; lifestyle changes. Kaitie did not think it was time for me to start taking a statin. Statins are incredibly common types of medication that block an enzyme that your liver produces that is required to create cholesterol. According to the CDC:

> Application of the 2018 Cholesterol Guideline to 2011–2018 NHANES data indicates that an estimated 46.1 million (M) US adults (19.9%) would be recommended statin use for cholesterol management
> Recommended and Observed Statin Use among U.S. Adults – National Health and Nutrition Examination Survey, 2011–2018[3]

It would be completely reasonable for a doctor to recommend a medication — particularly based on my cholesterol scores — but because she knows me and my obsessive-compulsive tendencies well enough, she figured we'd try some other things first. Here is what she suggested:

- Start intermittent fasting. She suggested that I go with five days a week and only eat between noon and 8 p.m.

- Normally, a doctor would suggest cutting out alcohol but because I already don't drink it (I've never liked the taste), this was an easy victory for me.

- Cut back on my soda intake.

- Reduce the amount of red meat I was eating.

---

[3] https://stacks.cdc.gov/view/cdc/127172#moretextPAmods.subject_name

- Start exercising more regularly.

Before I really knew how any of these things would go, it was important to me to understand why they were important. I do much better with a task if I understand the reasons why. Let's go into more detail on all these things and how they affect cholesterol. This is what I learned:

Intermittent fasting is commonly used by people as a way to lose weight. That may or may not work but was certainly not my goal. There were other potential benefits for me. My plan was to fast for 16 hours (8 pm until noon the next day). This does not include drinking water by the way (a great tip that worked for me while I was fasting and hungry was to just drink a bunch of water). After around 12 hours of fasting, your body will have depleted its glycogen stores (which we talked about earlier) and need to switch to burning fat for energy. Once you hit the 12-hour mark, there's a fancy word called *autophagy* that happens. Autophagy is made up of two Greek words: auto, which means "self" and phagy which means "eat." It is essentially the cleaning team in your body that breaks down damaged cell parts and therefore helps to maintain healthy cells. This in turn helps to reduce inflammation. Because your body isn't busy processing food your cells can focus more on cleaning up. The more cleanup, the less cholesterol, and the healthier the system.

Now for reduced soda intake. I decided that I would cut out soda entirely. Of course, nobody drinks soda, even the diet variety, and thinks they are drinking something healthy. However, I wanted to learn more about *why*. Here goes: When you drink soda, you're obviously consuming a ton of sugar; more than your body needs or can handle for energy production. This causes an insulin spike to handle the extra sugar. Your liver goes into overdrive to convert the extra sugar into triglycerides for storage because there's no other place to put it. Now you have more triglycerides in your blood and not enough HDL to clean it up. Also, your body is working to process that sugar so it can't be bothered to produce HDL. Because of the added insulin, your insulin sensitivity drops over time. It's a vicious cycle.

Red meat, burgers mostly for me, is a little more straightforward: Red meat is high in saturated fat. That fat directly raises the LDL (bad cholesterol). Red meat also has its own cholesterol just adding to the load.

Finally, add regular exercise. This is important for a number of reasons but as it relates to cholesterol, exercising increases your metabolic rate — it speeds up your body's engine. The faster your metabolism the better your body is at breaking down fats and using them for food. The exercise produces enzymes in your body that help to move the bad cholesterol (LDL) to your liver to be cleaned up while at the same time producing more of the good stuff (HDL). You then have more HDL to help with the general cleanup of the bad stuff. Exercise also reduces triglycerides by burning them directly for fuel. Exercise also improves insulin sensitivity which is good to help with fat management. It's a virtuous cycle.

Okay, so now I had things to try.

It was time to get to work. What happened next in this process ended up being a surprising and far greater adventure than I had expected. I learned more about myself — things I wasn't even aware I needed to learn — things that aren't even related to my physical health — than I had imagined. In the coming chapters, I'll not only explore what I did to change my life and how it worked (or didn't in some cases) but also how those things revealed facets of my personal nature I didn't know were there. I have discovered hidden insecurities, a lack of confidence, shame, pride, knowledge, awkwardness, and joy. I have discovered that accepting the situation and factors of my environment and life as "fine" or "normal" because "that's what happens as you get older" was not actually acceptable.

And so, it's time to get to work.

***

Something to think about...

What does being "fine" mean to you?

CHAPTER TWO

THE THIN MIRAGE

1

I thought the story began with a blood test in 2021, but that was just the climax of a much longer narrative. To understand how I spent decades confusing 'thin' with 'healthy,' we need to go back — way back — to when being called 'tiny' was just an observation, not a seed being planted.

I was born in the late 1970s but really grew up in the 1980s and the 1990s. I don't remember much from the 70s other than stories I've been told about the Blizzard of '78. I grew up in a suburb north of Boston, Massachusetts, called Peabody (pronounced pea-biddy — despite your desire to pronounce the way I know you want).

I was one of, if not the, shortest kid in my grade. I believe my pediatrician predicted, based on the way my height was trending, that I would end up being in the low end of the 5' range by the time I was finished growing. Throughout my youth, people felt the need to remind me, somewhat constantly, that I was "tiny." I never remember feeling bad about these comments but I certainly remember hearing them. Looking back now, there was likely some significance in terms of the impact it had on me, psychologically. I don't blame anyone. I didn't feel like I was being bullied. Being the shortest wasn't just a physical characteristic — it became part of my identity. People's constant need to comment on my size taught me early that bodies were something others felt free to discuss, judge, and categorize. At the time, I thought I was good with it. After all, it was just an objective fact — I was tiny. But looking back now, I realize these early experiences were laying the groundwork for something more complex.

While not underweight, probably because of my short stature, I was also regularly referred to as being very skinny. I was never in bad shape but I also never had what anyone would call good muscle tone.

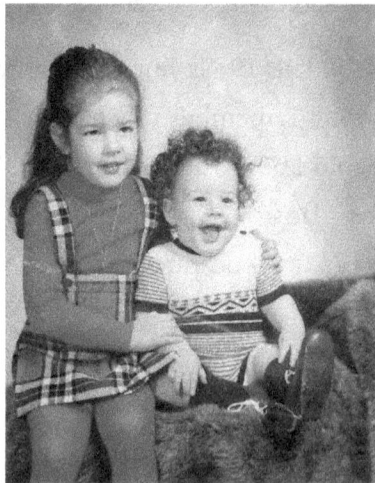

The picture above is of my sister and me. I was 15 years old at the time so you can see how tiny I looked. Oh, wait, that's not me as a 15-year-old. That's me as a baby. How about that hair? My sister and I still hold some deep-seated resentment towards our parents for dressing us up like we were trying to join the Von Trapp family. It doesn't matter that it was the 70s.

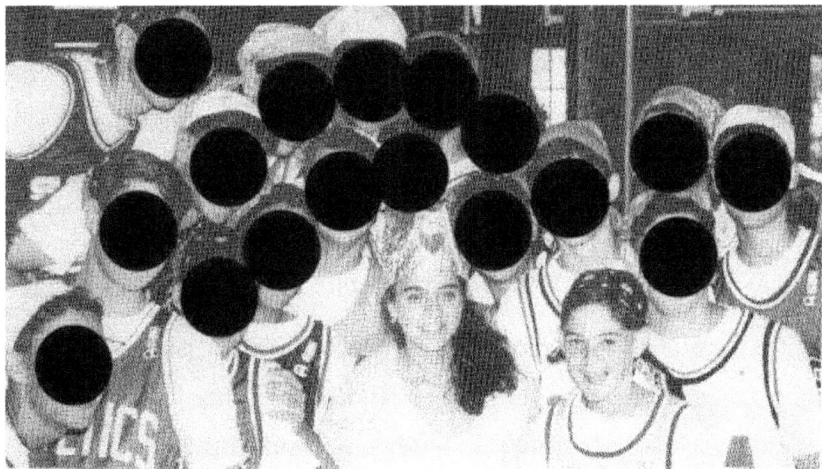

That's more like it. This is me, with the woman who would eventually become my wife (but not for a long time after this photo was taken). In this photo, I actually am 15. This photo is from the summer camp I attended as a kid. It comes from the last year I was a camper. That's right: the boy you see in the picture is part of the oldest group of campers. I was so close to the woman in the center (my now wife — jackpot for me — but that's a story for a different book) because this photo was taken at the end of an annual ceremony at camp where the oldest boy campers crown a "Queen," the youngest boy campers crown a "Princess," the youngest girl campers crown a "Prince," and the oldest girl campers crown a "King." The crowning happens after the group of campers marches around the dining hall singing parody songs giving hints as to who the person is going to be. The campers traditionally march in two columns, in height order with the shortest in front and the tallest in back. I'm next to her in the picture because I was first in line.

In each of the four years of my time in high school, I was elected to be the class treasurer. In each of those same years, there was a picture of the 4 officers in the school yearbook. I was the shortest one in three of those four pictures and then in my senior year, the growth spurt finally arrived. In that photo, I was the tallest. That year, when I was 17 turning 18, I grew almost an entire foot. This was significant for a few reasons:

1. I could reach the top cabinets.

2. What I didn't know then but do now is that growing that much in that short a period of time puts a lot of stress on your body and has not been wonderful for my body in the years since

3. I went from being tiny and skinny to tall and skinny and I had turned into what was referred to as a bean pole.

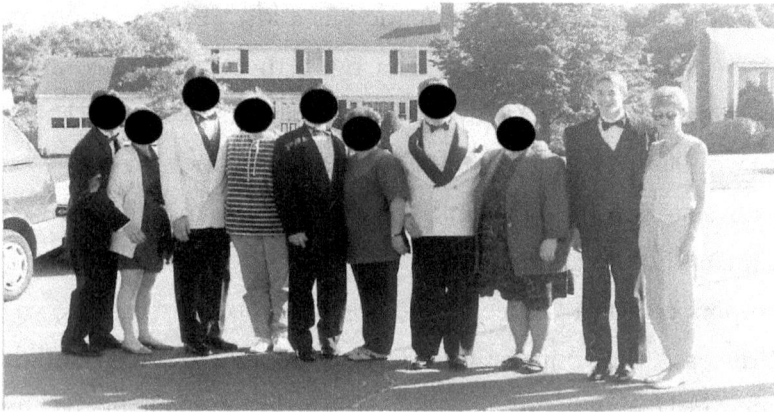

Before my senior prom with my mom. Now who's tall?

2

Then there were the sports. I played a lot of sports when I was a kid and news flash: I was good at them. I played Little League baseball and in various basketball leagues starting from a young age. On the baseball diamond, I started playing second base but pretty quickly moved to center field. I was not only a fast runner with good hand-eye coordination but in a bit of foreshadowing, I was really good at geometry. I was a natural at tracking the ball off the bat. Bonus: because I was so short when I played, it was nearly impossible to strike me out. Little League pitchers were generally not talented enough to thread the needle that was the *Matt Strike Zone*. I batted second and was an all-star table-setter. I stopped playing baseball when I started high school.

I did however continue to play basketball. I have always loved playing basketball. In that sport, I was a point guard which is the position often reserved for the smallest person on the team. I had a great outside shot and was good at facilitating the offense. I played on a variety of teams and when I got to high school, tried out for the freshman team. After tryouts, the coach pulled me aside and while I wish I was making this up, I'm not: he told me that I was not only really good and better than a lot of the people who tried out, I would not be making the team because I was too short. This was the first time I remember being actually angry about being called short.

I continued to play basketball on other teams and had a great time doing it. I never tried out for the high school basketball team again.

There was a high school team I did try out for, however: the tennis team. I played varsity tennis and more specifically, 1st doubles. To this day I still play tennis and still love it.

So I played and watched a lot of sports. I liked staying active. I was a nerdy kid who was also good at sports. This was befuddling for a lot of my friends. People often had a hard time reconciling this skinny but short-then-tall kid who was the class treasurer did tech work for the school theater, liked playing video games, was in the National Honor Society, loved Star Wars, Star Trek, The Golden Girls, and was also a really good athlete. I can't explain why this was so confusing for people but they did feel the need to let me know regularly.

To this day, when people find out that I not only enjoy playing sports but am good at them, they are shocked. I've never been able to figure out what it is about me that makes people assume that I couldn't or wouldn't want to do things that are athletic. Similarly, when COVID-19 was in its prime and we were all isolated in our homes, I, like most people who work, spent a lot of time in Zoom meetings. When I would eventually meet people in person, after having met them via virtual meeting, inevitably I'd get a comment like, "Wow, you're taller than I thought you'd be."

Maybe it's my personality. Maybe it's my head. Maybe it's IN my head.

3

Anyhow, what I haven't mentioned yet is how I always used to eat. Fast metabolisms run in my family. I got all the way into my 40s being able to eat anything I wanted, whenever I wanted, with no apparent effect. I also spent the majority of my life thinking I was a picky eater, and perhaps I am. It wasn't until relatively recently, maybe 5 or 6 years ago, that I figured out with a few smart co-workers that I was actually a super-taster[4].

A super-taster is someone who experiences taste much more intensely than the average person because they have more taste buds and more sensitive taste receptors on their tongues. Bitter foods like coffee or leafy greens are a hard pass. This is likely the reason I don't like alcohol. It's not that I'm picky but rather that I hate a lot of food and largely prefer basic foods like those found on the children's menus. While there's no direct correlation between super-tasters and people with high cholesterol, eating healthy vegetables is a great way to reduce cholesterol, and given that I'd rather poke my eyes out with an asparagus stalk than eat one, my dietary limitations haven't helped me.

When I was a kid I was either playing or watching sports every night. If it wasn't one of my games or matches, I would go watch my dad play on his softball or basketball teams. I loved doing that. After those games, we would almost always go to a local counter-order greasy take-out place. I would typically get chicken fingers, french fries, and a Coke or maybe I'd get a cheeseburger, French fries, and a Coke. This would often be at 9 pm or later. I have very fond memories of this part of my life.

I rarely ate any food that would be considered healthy unless you consider Drake's Devil Dogs to be healthy. I ate the food that I enjoyed. I was relatively active and through all that, my

---

[4] https://pmc.ncbi.nlm.nih.gov/articles/PMC3183330/

body never showed any signs of being anything other than fine. There was no abnormal weight gain or a big belly or anything like that. Chalk it up to a fast metabolism and onward we go.

My 'lucky' metabolism became both a blessing and a curse. Yes, I could eat anything without gaining weight, but this superpower came with an unexpected cost: it masked decades of unhealthy habits behind a thin facade. The super-taster revelation came years later, but it helped explain my limited food choices. While others might have been pushed toward healthier options by weight gain, my body never sent those signals. Being thin meant never having to question my choices — a freedom that would eventually catch up with me.

4

I attended college at Syracuse University and as might have been the case for you, college is the place where the concept of late-night eating is even more normalized. The number of times my roommate and I ordered Little Caesars or Domino's pizza after midnight would probably be considered *not ideal* in health circles. I wasn't even drunk. I was just hungry. With each pizza, there would also be a bottle of Coke. All the while, still being called skinny and still being considered as healthy. Through those years, once my height leveled off at 6'1" my weight pretty much stabilized as well and essentially didn't change for 20 years. No matter what I was doing in my life, including slowing down on the sports once I left high school, my weight stayed the same.

I think I know what you might be thinking: what a gift. Who wouldn't want to be skinny no matter what they eat and no matter what they do? I agree. It sounds great. It more than sounds great. It was great. I don't think I would go back in time, if I could, and change anything. My point here is that it became really easy to never think about my health because nothing I did ever affected my physical appearance and frankly, society told us that skinny was better. I appreciated how lucky I was.

I'm not blaming a single person for anything. I had a wonderful upbringing and so many great memories. I never felt like I was being bullied and I never felt bad about myself (although we'll explore in upcoming chapters how that may not have been the case). I'm not complaining about any of this. Rather, I'm on an expedition to look closely at my life prior to the moment when everything changed.

Being thin meant that people, including me, made assumptions solely based on my appearance and what they would see me eat. We all would equate my thinness and eating habits with being healthy. It must be so. Nobody ever questioned my food choices because "whatever you're doing must be working." After I left high school, I rarely exercised but it also didn't seem to matter.

"You must have the fastest metabolism!"

It turns out that after decades of living in this way, I developed blind spots. I never felt any external pressure to examine my habits. Again, I'm not blaming anyone. I am my own responsibility. Objectively, however, if you were in college and had a friend who was drinking every night, missing classes all the time, and stumbling around the dorm because they were drunk, at some point, you and other friends might intervene. If you saw enough behavior that you knew wasn't ideal and cared enough about the person exhibiting it, you'd probably try and help.

The problem was that nobody, including me, recognized any sort of problem then. I had a ton of friends and had a great time — even if it wasn't the same kind of raucous college time you see in the movies.

When college ended, I moved back to Massachusetts and started working immediately as a software engineer. I lived at home for 3 months before moving into an apartment with my best friend, who was my college roommate all through college and was ultimately the best man at my wedding. At this point, I was going for annual checkups at the doctor which would include blood work. As I mentioned in the previous chapter, my cholesterol was rarely perfect but was never considered concerning and certainly never bad.

5

This was around the time when I started experiencing back problems. In my youth, I had sprained both ankles multiple times (never both at the same time) which was about as much fun as you can imagine. The rapid growth during my senior year of high school was fun but set me up for a lifetime of weak joints. The back problems took me a long time to figure out. It started as "I'm not a kid anymore" and "maybe I just slept funny." Eventually, I started seeing a chiropractor and went for regular adjustments. These visits would help in the short term but never actually solved the problem. As a matter of fact, I didn't even know what the problem was. All I knew was that the chiropractor would tell me each time that my hips were out of alignment. I just resolved myself to the idea that I'd just have a bad back for the rest of my life.

After a few years of on-and-off back issues, my doctor recommended going to get an MRI and trying to find out what was going on. So I did. The MRI showed that one of my discs, probably the T5 or T6 (thoracic region) disc, was significantly smaller than the other discs. This created a weakness in the middle of my back. The hips being out of alignment would make me walk in an uneven way and that would put more pressure on my back. The recommendation was to start doing more exercise to strengthen my core. If I could protect my spine it would be less likely to give me issues.

This is around when I decided to go see a personal trainer at one of those boutique fitness places where you get 1-on-1 training. I found it to be a little bit interesting and a lot boring. The style was not for me and every time I would start to make any sort of progress I would have another issue with my back. These back spasms started happening more frequently and with more intensity and each time, it would mean I was not able to exercise for weeks after an incident. Those setbacks were pretty trying on me, particularly because I was still healthy according to my doctor at the time. I was still the right weight. I still looked the same with the exception of the occasional limp or hunch in my back depending on how I was feeling.

The next iteration of physical issues was when I felt a pop in the middle of my back. Did you know that your ribs are actually a kind of joint? If you aren't familiar with rib subluxation, you might want to sit down for this.

Maybe you don't think about this part of your body much but I definitely do…now. Imagine your rib cage and how it's mostly open in the front and connects to your spine in the back. The point where each rib connects to your spine is called a costovertebral joint. You know when you take a deep breath and your ribs expand? They are essentially pivoting open from your spine. If you have a muscle imbalance, poor core stability, repetitive strain, or maybe even a disc that's smaller than the others creating a weakness in that area, those joints could partially dislocate. It's the best time.

You know in the medical shows when the emergency room doctor pulls out the rib spreader device? That's what I imagine it feels like when my rib dislocates — but I'm awake. The pain is typically sharp and localized right around the dislocation. It becomes difficult to take any sort of deep breath and I pray that I won't need to cough or sneeze. I start to not want to move at all. When it would happen I would make an appointment with the chiropractor to pop it back in. The good news is that once it was back in, it would only be three or four weeks before it would feel normal again; all the while I'd be walking around on eggshells for fear of it happening again.

Each time a spasm or rib dislocation would happen it would require starting over on the exercise program and being even more careful so as to not create a bigger problem. I was never making any progress on the exercise (re: abs of steel) because I didn't have the time, knowledge, or experience to know what I was doing before I'd have another episode with my back. It started to seem like it wasn't worth the risk; particularly since I felt no sense of urgency given how ok I thought I was. This became another moment in my life to just settle for what was working and not push myself.

The back problems should have been my wake-up call. Instead, they became another thing to work around, another aspect of life to label as 'fine.' Each spasm, each rib dislocation was my body trying to tell me something I wasn't ready to hear. I was so accustomed to being 'naturally healthy' that I didn't recognize these issues as symptoms of a larger problem and not just 'getting older.'

Everything was fine.

6

Skip ahead to March of 2008.

At this point, I've been married for just over a year and my wife and my first daughter had been born. I have changed exactly zero of my food behaviors, play zero sports, and exercise zero days a week. I wrote a whole other book on my parenting experience called *Nature & Nurture: A Journey Through the Fog of Parenting*[5] so you can read all about that part of my life there. What's relevant here is that now I had added the activity of lifting and holding a baby, on one side. I had to actively try and switch sides from time to time so I wouldn't be quite as imbalanced. This was all well and good until April of 2009 when our second

---

[5] https://mattbrand.com/book

daughter was born. Now I was lifting and holding babies constantly. I was crouching and crawling and lifting and holding and squatting and laying down on floors and playing and running and up and down and over and out and in and around. It was non-stop movement with growing babies in both arms.

I started catching myself making grunts and groans when I was getting up from the floor and allowing gravity to assist me more when it was time to sit on the couch. It's ok though, I told myself, because this is what life is when you have babies. I just tried to be careful because if I had a back issue, or rather, when I had a back issue, that would make it really hard for me to help as much with our daughters.

The transition to parenthood brought new physical demands, but also new excuses. Those grunts and groans when getting up from the floor? Just part of being a dad. The increasing reliance on gravity to help me onto the couch? Normal aging. I had mastered the art of normalizing decline, all while maintaining the appearance of being 'healthy enough.'

Over all this time, I considered myself to be lucky to be thin. I still consider myself lucky that I was thin. Part of me wonders, though, had I been overweight, would I have been more likely to take my health seriously? I suspect the answer is yes. Please believe me when I say that I know this sounds like a "woe is me" type of problem. I'm not comparing my situation with anyone else's. I'm just suggesting, objectively and as a thought exercise, that if my circumstances were different, without judgment, would it have taken 44 years for me to really figure out that I needed to change the way I was living my life?

Of course, thought exercises are fun but not necessarily productive. Action is where the productivity comes from for me and so the only real question was, what happens next?

Looking back now, I can see how being naturally thin shaped not just my eating habits but my entire relationship with health. Being thin and getting used to others calling me 'skinny' created a blind spot so comfortable that it took forty-four years and a shocking blood test to finally see through it. The question wasn't just 'What happens next?' but 'How did I let it go so long?' The answer, I was learning, had less to do with metabolism and more to do with the stories I was telling myself about being 'fine.'

***

Something to think about...

What's one thing from your past that you would do differently if you knew then what you know now?

CHAPTER THREE

REASON TO CHOOSE

1

The first chapter described the problem I was facing. The second chapter described how I believe I got there. This chapter is about what transformed a shocking blood test into the catalyst for change.

For the briefest of moments, I thought, "I'm fucked."

But that moment passed quickly, replaced by something more powerful: the vision of all the moments I refused to miss.

When you see that your triglycerides are over 1000 and the optimal range is "anything under 150" it only takes a rudimentary understanding of math to know that you're way off. My number was seven times higher than the highest number in the ideal range. For me, this wasn't going to be just about one small change.

Once that brief moment passed there were a series of other moments to consider. I asked myself how possible it might be that I'd just keel over from a heart attack at any minute. For fun, I looked up what could happen if you have triglycerides over 1000:

- Acute pancreatitis is the most immediate danger. The pancreas becomes severely inflamed and can cause intense abdominal pain, vomiting, and life-threatening complications if not treated

- Huge risk of cardiovascular problems that could lead to a heart attack or a stroke

- Blood clots

- Fatty liver disease — in my case, this would technically be Non-Alcoholic Fatty Liver Disease or NAFLD for short. I won't go through all the symptoms but ultimately this can lead to liver failure.

What a party! As great as any of those sound, my preference was to have to deal with none of them. Seven times higher than the optimal range wasn't just a number — it was a warning shot across the bow of my future. Each potential complication represented moments I might miss and memories I might not get to make. The only option for me was to do what I could to mitigate as many of those risks as possible.

Resolved. I shall figure out what to do.

2

The next and biggest moment was: I am a husband and a father. I have responsibilities outside of myself. This was a real kick in the pants for me. I think it's normal, as one gets older, to accept that the way you are and the things that you can do change and potentially degrade as you age. When I was in college, regularly staying up until three in the morning eating pizza, and hanging out with friends was a ton of fun. I could just sleep the next day until dinner time. This would involve skipping breakfast and lunch but ultimately, it didn't matter. I felt great.

When I was younger my bones didn't creak like an old Victorian staircase and my joints didn't crackle and pop with every step I take like they do now. As I've mentioned, my metabolism was lightning fast and my body never changed — at least from what I, or anyone who knew me, could see — aside from getting tall during my senior year of high school.

As any of us get older, there are some pretty consistent physiological changes that we should be able to expect but generally don't think about until they happen. Related to muscle change, we will gradually lose muscle mass, lose strength, and have a harder time recovering. Our metabolism will decrease over time. Our bodies will store more fat. Our vision will deteriorate over time. Our blood vessels will get less flexible which will mean our blood pressure will go up and our hearts will have to work harder to do the same job. Our energy levels will go down and our bones will lose density. Does anything improve physically on its own as we get older? Unfortunately, I think the answer is no.

This is a grim picture to paint but is a reality for all people regardless of *other* medical conditions someone might be dealing with. The cholesterol problem I was now facing was in addition to the standard set of age-related changes that were inevitably coming my way.

I like to think that I'm a generally unselfish person most of the time — but not all the time. I'm sure other people have had similarly really bad cholesterol and decided that whatever happens, happens; that the changes required to improve a health situation might not be worth it to someone or might be too difficult. If not for my family's presence in my life, I don't know if I'd have been as motivated to do everything I could to improve my health.

Months before my fateful doctor's appointment in July of 2021, my father had his own health issues. Watching him experience those followed shortly after by my results, albeit less acutely severe than his, was a little like looking at a crystal ball and seeing your future. I started thinking about all the things that I wanted to experience with my daughters. They were 12 and 13 years old at the time with so much life ahead of them and so many things that I *NEEDED* to be there to see.

It wasn't just about being alive — it was about being present. Really present. Not the dad who has to sit out the games, or watch the graduations from the back because he can't walk to the front, or miss the wedding dance because his heart can't take it. I started listing all the moments I refused to miss.

There was going to high school and getting drivers licenses and going on college visits and high school graduations and college drop-offs and parents weekends at college and drunk calls in the middle of the night from college and college graduations and career searches and first jobs and moving home (fingers crossed) and run-on sentences and meeting partners and weddings to plan and weddings to attend and dances to have and speeches to make and finding out you're going to be a grandfather and then finding our you're going to be a grandfather again and helping to build a crib and doing a terrible job of painting a nursery and meeting your first grandchild and then meeting your second grandchild and babysitting for your grandchildren and watching your grandchildren try to eat cake on their first birthdays and watching your grandchildren walk for the first time and babysitting your grandchildren for a week while their parents go on vacation and seeing pictures of their first day of school and going to watch them perform in the 3rd grade production of The Music Man and writing letters to them when they go to sleep-away camp and being there for elementary school graduation and watching middle school volleyball games and going to their b'nai mitzvahs and seeing them go to high school and waiting for them to inevitably ignore me because they have friends they'd prefer to hang out with and talking to them about their moms' college searches and feeling so excited to find out they were going to college and watching them graduate from high school and getting drunk calls in the middle of the night because they thought they were dialing one of their parents and being able to attend their college graduations and being wheeled into their weddings and getting to hold my great grandchildren.

These are all things I decided I couldn't miss to the extent that I had any control. There are, of course, factors outside of my control but for those that I could, I would. I wanted to make sure that I wasn't just alive for as long as possible — which clearly was limited with the approach I had been taking — but that I was able to have as healthy a life as possible. I don't want to sound presumptuous and assume that anyone else, my daughters included, needs me to be around (although I'd like to think they'd say that). I wanted to make sure that at the very least they had the option of having me around and healthy. Yes, there is definitely some selfishness baked into this along with a reasonable amount of self-delusion. My idea of what my daughters and wife need is less relevant than their own ideas. I don't speak for them but I have to believe — please let me be right — that their world is better with me in it and it's even better if I'm healthy.

There is of course no guarantee and no crystal ball on any of this. There's a non-zero, but probably low, chance that if I had changed nothing, I could get lucky and still be around for all of the things that will eventually happen in my daughters' lives. I could go to a casino and throw some money in a slot machine or some chips on the craps table and I might lose a little and then win a little and then lose some more. I could end up gambling for a long time and keep telling myself that the next pull of the slot arm or the next roll of the dice will be the big win and so I should keep going. I could also choose to take my winnings or even what I have left and walk away from the table and walk away from the machine and figure out a way to re-invest what I have left into something that has better odds of being productive.

3

Have you heard the concept of healthspan vs lifespan? This is another concept that Dr. Peter Attia discusses in "Outlive: The Science & Art of Longevity" and is covered in a variety of other places. Basically, lifespan refers to the number of years someone is alive from birth until death. Healthspan refers to the number of years where someone does not have a significant illness or disease. You can read an interesting article about why healthspan could be more important than lifespan in Time magazine[6] from November of 2023.

Essentially, I asked myself if I would rather live to be 95 years old but spend the final years of that dealing with a plethora of ailments while being miserable, or would I prefer to live to be 85 years old and be happy and healthy? I understand it's not a simple question and is more of a philosophical debate. This raises a different question: what if I can maximize both? In order for me to experience all the things I want to experience and be around the people in my life for whom I care and who I hope also care about me, what I really need is time. I can't guarantee how that time will be spent but I can guarantee that it was time to commit to doing everything I could do to make sure I was in the best possible position to survive with an abundance of happiness and an age-appropriate amount of health for as long as possible.

Regardless of the cholesterol situation I was dealing with, there is plenty of data about the correlation between people who

---

[6] Why 'Healthspan' May Be More Important Than Lifespan:
https://time.com/6341027/what-is-healthspan-vs-lifespan/

take preventative health measures and their longevity. For example, people who partake in regular moderate exercise — at least 2 1/2 hours per week — reduce all-cause mortality by 30-40%. Just go for a brisk walk a few times a week. Strength training helps build and maintain muscle mass and bone density (which we know deteriorates over time). Balancing exercises are good to help minimize the risk of falling as you get older. Getting seven to eight hours of quality sleep each night is good to support metabolic health. Poor sleep contributes to the risk of cardiovascular disease and cognitive decline. The amount of data and choices that are available could fill up a shopping mall. You don't have to choose to do everything but any one thing you choose to do reduces your risk and increases the likelihood of a long and healthy life.

And even the smallest iterative improvements have a compounding benefit over time. Let's use walking as an example. Let's say you are committed to going for a 15-minute walk, twice a day. As I mentioned, moderate exercise for 2 1/2 hours per week, or 150 minutes, is a great goal. If you do two 15-minute walks a day for five days and take the other two days off, you've reached the goal of 150 minutes. Here are some of the benefits of those walks:

In the short term, you will be in a better mood because of the endorphin release from taking the walk. Your blood sugar regulation will be improved if you take a walk after meals. You will sleep better, and your blood pressure will drop for 24-48 hours after the walk. After the first few months of that, you'll start to reap bigger benefits: your heart muscle will start to strengthen along with your leg muscles and your general sense of balance. Your insulin sensitivity will improve along with your immune system. Generally, your cardiovascular fitness will improve. If you continue with this routine beyond a year you will likely be lowering the risk of getting type 2 diabetes, reducing the risk of acquiring heart disease, and may even get cognitive benefits like reducing the risk of dementia.

And there are other intangible benefits as well: walking with a friend. This is a social benefit and it's a great chance to connect with someone. It's also a great excuse to take a break from whatever it is you're doing — a break you deserve — which in turn can reduce your stress. Chronic stress will increase the rate of your cellular aging. In my opinion, there is an even bigger benefit. Walking, or whatever you choose to do for your moderate exercise is a gateway to adding other healthy habits.

4

As we'll explore in upcoming chapters, once you start a healthy habit and see some form of a positive result — which you will if you walk regularly — you will likely be much more open and interested in adding other healthy habits to your repertoire. This is called habit stacking.

There is a common framework for habit formation. It has four stages and goes a little something like this:

1. Cue: this is the trigger that causes your brain to initiate action.

2. Craving: this is the motivation to change.

3. Response: this is the action or set of actions that you take to actually do something.

4. Reward: this is the satisfaction — the prize — for doing something from the previous step. This reward can then become the cue for the next round.

There's a great article from James Clear called "How To Start Habits That Actually Stick[7]" that does a great job of explaining the loop. There are a few basic concepts that need to be true for these steps to actually turn into a habit and loop; to continue. From his article:

> Eliminate the cue and your habit will never start. Reduce the craving and you won't experience enough motivation to act. Make the behavior difficult and you won't be able to do it. And if the reward fails to satisfy your desire, then you'll have no reason to do it again in the future. Without the first three steps, a behavior will not occur. Without all four, a behavior will not be repeated.
> James Clear, "How To Start Habits That Actually Stick"

Each of us has different things that motivate us in our lives. I'm the kind of person who loves learning about as much as possible. I want to know how things work and then seek out the answers. Related to that, I need to know the reason for doing something before I do it and I'm also hyper-competitive although I'm not entirely sure that the people who know me the best know that. For me, the desire to learn how things work and

---

[7] How To Start Habits That Actually Stick by James Clear: https://jamesclear.com/three-steps-habit-change

my generally competitive nature mean that when I set my mind on a goal, it's going to happen.

I also have the ability to be very patient. I've been willing to put the work in to get better at something as I learn more about it. Understanding the science of habit formation wasn't just academic — it was my roadmap to being there for every moment I wanted to experience. Each stage of the habit loop was another step toward the future I wanted. If I apply the habit formation framework to my own situation, here is how it would look:

1. Cue: the first cue should be pretty obvious — getting a call from your doctor telling you that you have cholesterol that's dangerously high

2. Craving: this whole chapter is about the craving to change. Primarily for me, it's my family. I had to be better for them.

3. Response: this is what I'll start to explore in the coming chapters.

4. Reward: I'm writing this book so you can be reasonably sure that I didn't die right away. The reward, it turns out, was not — and has not been — what I expected it to be. I will also go into that in the coming chapters. What I can tell you, however, is that the reward, or rewards, have been far more fulfilling and far more motivational than I could have imagined and more than enough motivation to repeat the cycle.

I don't want to spoil what's coming later in the book but I'll give you the tiniest tease: I think given the problem that I was presented with and that you've read about, you could assume that if I just made some dietary changes and did some exercise, my cholesterol levels would drop and I'd have better heart health. Maybe I'd end up in better shape. Maybe I'd have better energy. Maybe I'd sleep better or feel less stressed.

If those were the only outcomes — the only rewards if you will — I'd consider myself to be very lucky and for this journey to have been a success. The good news is, I learned a lot more about a lot more than I thought I would. I found more things to be passionate about and a better reason to prioritize the things that are important to me.

Everyone has a choice. Please believe me when I say this: there is no judgment here. You don't have to agree with me or follow the same path. You don't have to be motivated by the things that motivate me. You do have to decide what your motivation is and if that motivation, that craving, is strong enough to decide to do things in different ways than what you're used to doing. It is not easy to decide to change and it's even harder to actually change. The good news: once you get that first reward for your hard work, it does get easier to continue to change.

Ultimately, my health is my responsibility and nobody else's. When I was growing up, nobody told us how bad cigarettes were for you. I didn't blame anyone for smoking. As a matter of fact, society was told that cigarettes were cool. Over time, we — as in people who aren't Big Tobacco — learned that cigarettes were in fact not good for you. Once the inputs change, your context changes and so can your outputs.

I don't look back with regret at the choices that led to that blood test. Those choices were made by a different version of me, operating with different information. But now I had new information, new motivation, and a choice to make: would I accept the life that was happening to me, or choose the life I wanted to create? The answer would determine not just my future, but the quality of countless moments with the people I love most.

Once I knew differently, that was the moment to make a choice. I have people who count on me. I have people I count on. I want them to do everything they can to be the best versions of themselves and it would not be fair to ask that of them if I wasn't willing to do the same for myself. So I ask you this: are you going to comfortably sit back and accept the way life is or do you want to lean forward and choose the way your life is going to be?

***

Something to think about...

What future moments do you want to be present and healthy for?

PART TWO

CHOOSING CHANGE

CHAPTER FOUR

THE FIRST STEP

1

July 20, 2021

I hung up the call with Kaitie.

For me, this wasn't about new beginnings — those tend to fade. This was about methodical change. As a software engineer, I approach problems systematically: understand the why, establish measurable goals, implement solutions, and test results. My body had presented me with a bug to fix, and I needed to debug it properly.

This isn't intended to be preachy or prescriptive. The goal here is to share the steps I took but hopefully through a lens that helps you to better understand your own options. Also, just because one thing or another worked well (or didn't work well) for me doesn't mean that you would have the same outcome.

Figure your own shit out. Maybe you can use my shit to help guide yours.

Like in my professional life as a software engineer, the first thing I have to be comfortable with before I start building that next feature or fixing a bug is the why of it all. I have to understand the actual problem I'm trying to solve. The way we each define our goals may be quite different. For me, I need to be able to objectively define the desired outcome, and the more things I can measure that help me feel comfortable that I'm on the right track, the better. I'm not wonderful at jumping into a void of the unknown and seeing where it takes me.

For me, there was one initial and measurable goal I was after: get my triglyceride number down to at least 150. That's it. That was my North Star. Everything that I was about to do was in service of that single goal. I had no plan or intention to lose weight or sleep better or feel better or even get in shape. If any or all of those things also happened, as side effects, that would be a bonus. If by the next time my blood was tested my triglycerides had gone down, I knew that I'd feel like I was making progress with whatever I was doing and would keep on going. I am motivated by results.

Goals, for me, should be aspirational but not so much so that they aren't attainable. Goals can change. They can evolve.

2

I had resolved myself to try a few things. In hindsight and in particular as someone who appreciates science, how things work, and measurable outcomes, it probably would have been more instructive for me to do one of the following things at a time so I could see how each affected me. In any scientific experiment — and that's what this would be — it is better to test one variable at a time. The moment you start testing multiple variables that could affect each other, it gets much harder to know which variable is producing which outcome.

Alas, I can't go back. The next blood test would be in September of 2021, just two months later.

Intermittent Fasting

Kaitie had suggested that I start intermittent fasting. She had suggested that even if I did it 4 or 5 days a week, only eating between noon and 8 pm on those days, it could make a huge difference. I explained the science of intermittent fasting in the first chapter so I won't repeat that here. I decided — given my obsessive-compulsive tendencies and my love of routines — that I would do intermittent fasting 7 days a week. I figured it would be easier for me to do that than it would be to have different eating schedules on different days. Also, given that I had a habit of eating pretty late at night from time to time, restricting any eating to the chosen feeding window seemed like a better approach for me. I would begin immediately.

Given my high metabolism, I figured it would take some time for my body to adjust to intermittent fasting. The good news is that it only took a few days of body confusion before I started being less hungry at times when I used to eat. The bad news: it turned out I didn't fully understand how to do it. At first, I treated intermittent fasting as a practice of essentially cutting out breakfast and late-night snacks. I was effectively eating 1/3 —

from a caloric perspective — of what I had been eating for the first 44 years of my life. On the fateful July 20 visit of 2021, I weighed 166 pounds. On the next visit, which was two months later on September 16, 2021, I weighed 153 pounds. That's roughly 8% of my body weight in what was just slightly under 2 months. Like I've said, I wasn't overweight but was now trending towards being underweight. I was simply not eating enough calories given this style of time-restricted eating in combination with the other things I had started (and stopped) doing.

Eventually, I figured out that I had to essentially eat the same volume of food I was eating before but do so in a smaller window of time. It took me some time to work that out though. On December 20, 2021, I had my second follow-up appointment, and that time I weighed 149 pounds and my BMI had dropped to 19.7. The acceptable range of BMI for a man my age at the time was anywhere between 19 and 26.9. My BMI when this started, on July 20 of 2021 was 21.95.

Back then, I treated BMI like some sort of mystical number that doctors used to judge me. It wasn't until later that I understood what it really meant: Body Mass Index is a simple calculation dividing your weight in kilograms by your height in meters squared. It is a basic metric that doesn't account for muscle mass, bone density, gender, or age.

So now I had created a new problem. I was losing weight fairly drastically; something I didn't want to do.

Now take a little step back before we get on to the next thing. Intermittent fasting can be a dietary mechanism that people use for losing weight but that is — and was for me — because of a decline in caloric intake. I didn't lose weight specifically because I was only eating in an 8-hour window. I was losing weight because I wasn't eating enough. As a matter of fact, if you were to choose to try intermittent fasting, I'd caution you to really understand its implications before you get started. Because you aren't eating for long periods of time, you might find yourself feeling pretty low energy. Depending on how you typically spend your days, you may not be able to afford to have low energy. This low energy could lead to difficulty concentrating, low attention spans, and mood swings.

Also, if you take medications that are required at specific times of the day, depending on when those times are, intermittent fasting might not be right for you. Any amount of caloric intake outside the fasting window will end the fast. You heard me Mr. coffee with anything in it[8]. Also, fasting doesn't really start until after your body is finished digesting. I was making sure I stopped eating by 8 pm (but usually earlier than that) so that by the time I got into bed, my body was done "working." To reiterate, intermittent fasting was never about losing weight for me; it was about that fancy *autophagy* word from Chapter 1 where my body would essentially start eating itself, starting with the bad stuff.

Soda

As of July 20, 2021, I have not had any soda. I stopped drinking it; cold turkey. As an expansion of that, at that moment I also essentially stopped drinking anything that wasn't water. This included things like orange juice — which I was a big fan of

---

[8] I don't drink coffee and never have but I'm told it's a fairly popular beverage in adult humanity.

in the morning. I always appreciated water but was never a huge water drinker; probably because I drank so much soda and that was my preference. For example, if I went out to see a movie at the theater, it would be a huge Coca-Cola. From that day, the huge Coca-Cola became a bottle of water. Since that day, my appreciation for water has increased by a ton (cold water in particular). At first, I thought I would get bored of it or miss the taste of soda.

Recently one of my daughters asked me if I ever got the urge to drink soda. I told her that not only had I not gotten the urge to drink it, I was fairly certain I wouldn't even like it. If you knew me prior to 2021, this would likely be something shocking to hear. I have specifically avoided soda water, ginger ale, or anything carbonated because I was nervous that this style of beverage would make me want to drink Coca-Cola again.

65.

That is the number of grams of sugar in one 20oz bottle of Coke. That is the equivalent of 16.25 teaspoons of sugar. To put that into perspective, according to the American Heart Association[9], men should consume no more than 9 teaspoons of added sugar per day. NINE. Women should consume no more than 6 teaspoons of sugar in a day. No big deal. As a caveat, these numbers don't include naturally occurring sugars like those found in fruit. A single 20oz bottle of Coca-Cola Classic, my

---

[9] American Heart Association's Daily Sugar intake:
https://www.heart.org/en/healthy-living/healthy-eating/eat-smart/sugar/how-much-sugar-is-too-much#:~:text=Men%20should%20consume%20no%20more,or%20100%20calories)%20per%20day.

favorite of the Coca-Colas had almost twice the recommended daily limit. Let's also say that on an average day, I drank at least two — if not more — bottles of Coke. Just typing it here makes me cringe. Even if that was the only sugar intake for me I am imagining spooning 32 teaspoons of sugar into my mouth, every day. The bad news: it wasn't the only sugar I was ingesting.

Water, on the other hand, has 0 grams of sugar. Drink as much as you'd like. What should seem obvious but was never something I thought about before was how good water is for you. Not just for hydration but for kidney function and better digestion, among other things. If you treat it like a substitute for soda, now you're talking about reducing caffeine dependency, not having as many artificial additives/sweeteners, and not damaging your teeth.

Before you ask — yes — I know Diet Coke doesn't have sugar in it. It does however have a lot of other things in it that aren't great for you with the most commonly discussed ingredient of aspartame. Aspartame can cause headaches, anxiety, weight gain (irony), cardiovascular issues, and others. Diet Coke definitely has less sugar than regular Coke but still isn't a healthy drink. It's a lot of flavored chemicals.

Exercise

The goal was to start exercising — as a deliberate choice — regularly. This can be a daunting task for anyone because at the beginning it feels like there are an infinite amount of things you *could* do but you might be unclear on what you *should* do. Later on in the book, I'll spend more time talking specifically about the things I've learned about exercise through this journey but for now, let's discuss the basics.

There are typically two high-level types of exercise that I think most people are familiar with: cardiovascular training (cardio) or strength training (lifting weights). Both provide different types of benefits. As someone who grew up playing sports and is now an adult human, I figured I could stick to the basics: go for some runs in the neighborhood and do some crunches, or something. I had no equipment in my house for either cardio or strength training other than a Peloton bike I was using from time to time. We had that bike because I thought it would be good to have. This was one of those, "I'll use it if I pay for it" types of situations. I figured I'd just start moving my body a bit. This is, of course, better than not moving your body a bit.

Cardiovascular training brings with it a series of benefits. It strengthens your heart and lungs and can burn more calories during the actual exercise which is great if you're trying to lose weight and are less concerned or interested in building muscle. Weight — by the way — in overly simplistic terms goes up if you consume more calories than you burn off and goes down if you burn more calories than you consume. Because cardio strengthens your heart and lungs, it increases your stamina. As it relates to cholesterol management, cardio directly raises your HDL levels (which is great) and again, because it strengthens your heart, your blood flow improves which is good for fighting cholesterol by being better at metabolizing fats into energy.

Strength training is great for building and maintaining muscle. It can also increase your bone density. Because you have stronger muscles, your metabolism improves which is good for burning more calories even when you're at rest (as opposed to cardio which will burn more calories while you're in the exercise itself). Strength training is also good for functional strength, like balance and grip strength. Additionally, it can improve joint stability which is especially good for people who grew way too much in a short period of time when they were seniors in high school and have dealt with *challenging* joint issues since then. Also, it's natural and expected to lose muscle mass as you get older so the more you pack on now the better you are setting yourself up for later. Cholesterol you ask? That lean muscle mass that you're adding means better glucose regulation and better handling of fat in your body. Results can take longer to show with strength training but are likely to last longer.

Both cardio and strength training also just feel good because they both release endorphins. I don't know about you but I have known the word "endorphin" and what it generally meant but never really understood it. They are natural hormones that your body produces that reduce pain perception and make you feel good. What I learned pretty quickly — even if I wasn't entirely sure of what I was doing — is that exercising was energizing. On days when I wouldn't exercise, I noticed a significant change in my energy levels for that day. If I really think hard about this, and I am, I am sure that some of that energy stemmed from the mental satisfaction of exercising. It felt like I was achieving something towards my goal of getting healthier. Even if I didn't exactly know how to measure my progress yet, in my mind, at least I was trying.

According to the American Heart Association[10], getting 2.5 hours of moderate-intensity aerobic (cardio) exercise per week and at least 2 days a week of strength training is recommended. You can substitute the 2.5 hours of moderate cardio with 75 minutes of intense cardio if you'd prefer. Generally, I knew I wanted to do some of each. So that's what I did. It was the summer when this journey began for me so going for light runs outside a few days a week and then also doing what I thought might be considered a strength-training workout at home a few days a week as well.

3

I remember the first few days of this — feeling quite motivated — and thinking, "This is totally working." I'm fairly certain the feeling of success was mostly from the act of doing *something* as opposed to what I had been doing until then: *nothing*. I remember feeling excited to go to the local sporting goods store and buy myself some exercise shirts I could wear while running and working out. This was an indication to myself that I was serious about what I was doing. I remember thinking, after perhaps a week of this new exercise routine, that if I just kept it up for another few weeks I'd probably not only have much more muscle tone but also that my bad cholesterol would melt away. That — I figured — was how exercising worked. If you just do it for a few weeks you'll reach all your goals.

---

[10] American Hearth Association's Recommendations for Physical Activity in Adults and Kids: https://www.heart.org/en/healthy-living/fitness/fitness-basics/aha-recs-for-physical-activity-in-adults

I suspect this was my version of what I'll call "The New Year's Resolution Conundrum." According to the Pew Research Center, most New Years resolutions are related to health, exercise, or diet[11]. Many people say they have goals — they want to lose weight, they want to gain muscle, they want to look a certain way, etc. Often times though, people don't stick to those resolutions. This often happens because we set unrealistic goals (i.e. I want to lose 30 pounds by February or I want a six-pack by the summer). When you don't see immediate results towards your goals, you're more likely to decide that the effort isn't working and bail on it. Because you are new to it (I was), you probably aren't capable of setting realistic expectations (I wasn't) and therefore you are more likely than not going to disappoint yourself. Disappointment is rarely a good motivator to keep doing something. Also, unless you're a professional (foreshadowing for me) in the goal area, it is really hard to have a well-defined and well-informed action plan. We also don't always have a good support system or someone to hold us accountable for these goals. We are social creatures — even an extroverted-introvert like me — and having someone to talk to about the journey and the goals is really helpful. When you're new to a routine or trying to form a positive habit like exercising regularly, you may not know how to properly track progress (I didn't). All of these things contribute to the risk of losing motivation. If you don't feel like you're making any sort of progress because you aren't tracking it or nobody is talking to

---

[11] Pew Research Center on New Years resolutions:
https://www.pewresearch.org/short-reads/2024/01/29/new-years-resolutions-who-makes-them-and-why/

you about it or simply because life and all the other responsibilities you have gets in the way, you're much more likely to just tell yourself that you'll try again later — even if you and I both know that you probably won't.

Starting a positive habit — either as part of a New Year's Resolution or any other time of the year — is not dissimilar to working at tech startups (like I've done for the majority of my career). You have a great idea and the best intentions but the reality is, most of the time those companies fail. They fail for any number of reasons; some of which are controllable and some aren't. When (and I hope yours doesn't) the company fails, you move on to the next great idea and the next set of best intentions.

We'll come back to exercise shortly but before we do, let's cover the last big change area I was taking on:

Diet

Someone once asked me if was more of an "eat to live" type of person or a "live to eat" type of person. I've always considered myself to be in the former group. I enjoy food but I'm definitely not a foodie. I also don't have what anyone would consider to be a broad palate of food interests. Give me a chicken parm and ziti any day of the week. Actually, give me a chicken parm and ziti every day of the week. Actually, I'll take a burger on all those days too. The basics have always been fine for me. As I mentioned in the second chapter, I'm a super-taster. For many years I just assumed I was a picky eater. I should perhaps recategorize that though: I just assumed I was *only* a picky eater. Part of why I don't partake in a wide variety of different foods is because so many of the commonly eaten foods taste like garbage to me. I'm not judging broccoli or anything but I can barely stand the smell of it let alone the taste. That has always and also been the case for most other green foods. You may not be aware of this but those types of foods are commonly categorized as something called a "vegetable." Fortunately, both of my daughters have enjoyed vegetables.

Because I didn't eat those, with the exception of the widely accepted "best vegetable" that goes by the name of iceberg lettuce (the mostly unknown and unaccepted *leaf state* of water), I wasn't getting a lot of nutrients my body needed for general health. I was eating a ton of red meat and a fair amount of sugar (beyond the tons of sugar from soda). I was also eating a lot of late-night food (which was addressed with intermittent fasting).

My goal with my diet was pretty modest: replace some of the less desirable stuff with more desirable stuff. I also wanted to try to introduce some new foods into my diet that I had never liked before. I have gone through various cycles of "maybe if I just force myself to eat broccoli enough I'll condition myself to like it." There are videos of me trying a piece of broccoli and then almost passing out from disgust. That strategy has never proven to be viable for me. I stopped eating fast food burgers and when out at a restaurant, stopped defaulting to a burger and instead introduced something like a Caesar salad with grilled chicken. I had never been a huge fan of grilled chicken before or even Caesar salad but it turns out, this old dog could learn a new trick. I started to really like that and it became my new default. While Caesar salad dressing is not incredibly healthy for you, having that with the grilled chicken was — for me — a big improvement from constant burgers.

This is around the time when I started to learn about macros and went back to the exercise point about being able to track progress. I wanted to start learning and being mindful about what I was actually putting into my body. I'm not a nutritionist but learned the basics about macros.

The main types of macronutrients (macros) that people talk about are proteins, carbohydrates, and fats. Protein is what your body uses to build and repair muscle tissues. It is good for creating enzymes and hormones and supports your immune system. Meat, fish, poultry, eggs, and Greek yogurt are good natural sources of protein. Carbohydrates (carbs) are your body's primary energy source. They fuel your brain function and having enough carbs means your body can use those, and not protein, for energy. Whole grains like rice and quinoa along with fruits, potatoes, beans, and pasta are all good sources of carbohydrates. Finally, fats are what your body uses to store energy. The fats also protect your organs and help to absorb vitamins. Foods like avocados, nuts, salmon, and eggs are good sources of healthy fat.

In the beginning, I didn't have any specific macro goals. I not only didn't know enough about their value but didn't want to create too much work for myself at the beginning. Remember, this was a lighter and hopefully more easily attainable goal: just make incremental improvements to my diet and have a slightly better understanding of how nutrition works. I decided I would introduce yogurt into my diet. I was never a big fan but perhaps if I could find the right flavor and texture it would be a good replacement snack for some of the junk I was eating. I tried a variety of brands and generally liked most of them, and now we have a dedicated drawer in the refrigerator for yogurt. It has become my go-to snack. It's not only that the yogurt I was (and am) eating is high in protein but it's also satiating. Subtracting the negative effects of the junk I was eating alone was an improvement. Adding in the positive effects of something like yogurt and it's a double-win for me.

To recap, I started intermittent fasting to encourage my body to start doing some heavy lifting on my behalf to attack the bad cholesterol from the inside. I cut out soda to drastically reduce my sugar intake and drastically reduce the amount of extra sugar my body didn't know what to do with. I started exercising in order to build muscle and increase my good cholesterol. I made small and incremental improvements to the way I was eating by replacing some of the less-good food with more actual-good food.

This is where the fun really started.

***

Something to think about...

What's one small thing you can do today to improve your health?

CHAPTER FIVE

HIDDEN REFLECTIONS

1

S poiler alert: this is the chapter where I'll cover a topic that I didn't see coming. There are some other things to cover first but when I finished the outline for this book, this was the chapter that I had the most difficult time wrapping my head around. I've spent more time trying to figure out how to write about the topics in this chapter than any of the others and I think, when you get there, you'll understand why. That I've spent so much time trying to work through the right way to communicate what's on my mind is further proof of what I have discovered about myself and what I've been dealing with. Let's begin.

When I started on my quest to get healthier I did so by essentially just jumping in; head first. I decided that I would figure it out as I went along. I was trying to not look too far into the future. I knew I had a follow-up appointment in September of 2021, a mere two months later. I was hoping that I would see some sort of progress. In my head, I decided that while I was now doing intermittent fasting, had cut out all soda, and was eating incrementally better, those changes would be much harder to measure on my own in those two months. In my head, I figured that the exercise was where I'd see the biggest improvement and I felt like I needed to see some sort of change to feel like I was at least on the right path. I'm not sure I had a specific and measurable goal in mind given that I was just piecing together my exercise routine on my own. I did not tell myself that by the time the appointment rolled around my biceps would grow by a certain amount or that I would lose 10 pounds. I was just "asking" for any sign of progress. I told myself that this would be the validation I needed to keep going.

So YouTube became my friend. I started looking up exercises I could do at home. I wanted to be very careful because of my history of back problems. I started to do things that I thought might be helpful. I neither thought about nor cared about proper form. All you have to do is do some squats and do some sit-ups and some jumping jacks and go for a few jogs a week and voila, you're a bodybuilder! During that time, I don't remember ever feeling surprised when I caught a glimpse of myself in the mirror as if things were working so well but I was also pleased with myself for staying committed to the concept of exercise. In addition to the runs I would go for outside, I was starting to ride the Peloton bike a bit more often. I thought things were going pretty well — which they were — relatively.

The first step is to take the first step and that's what I had done.

2

September 16, 2021, 7:00am

I walked into the doctor's office for my appointment with Kaitie. I was pretty excited to be there and not only fill her in on all the changes I had made but even more excited to get my blood drawn so I could see what my latest cholesterol numbers looked like. Even in a world where after 2 months you *could* have transformed your body into the best physical condition of its life, you'd still have no way of knowing what was going on with your cholesterol without the blood test. I filled Kaitie in on all that was going on but the only physical change that was discernible was my weight. I was now 153 pounds. That meant that I had lost 13 pounds — 8% of my body weight — since the previous appointment in July. There was no real visible change to the composition of my body. The conversation with Kaitie ended and it was time for my aforementioned outstanding veins to do their thing. The nurse came in and took my blood. Later that day, I got the results:

September 2021 Bloodwork Results

Measure	Result	Optimal Range
Total Cholesterol	201	140-200
Calculated LDL	109	0-129, <100 optimal
Cardiac Risk	5.6	0-5
Triglycerides	282	<150 optimal
HDL	36	>40 optimal
Non-HDL	165	---

My total cholesterol number was now just outside the optimal range, down to 201 from 247. My cardiac risk dropped from 6.9 in July down to 5.6. This is still outside the optimal range but had dropped almost 20%. My HDL score did not change at all. The number that gave me a moment to celebrate though was the triglycerides. That number went from 1036 down to 282. That's a nearly 73% drop in a pretty short amount of time.

Things were working. I was really pleased with myself. I guess I could just keep doing what I was doing and hope things trended in the right direction. My next appointment was scheduled for December, 3 months later.

After I read those results I was even more motivated. This was the proof I needed to *know* that whatever I was doing — regardless of whether it was the intermittent fasting, the removal of soda from my life, the improved eating, the exercise, or the likely combination of all of them — had set me on a path to getting healthy. It was an incredible feeling and this is when my competitive nature really kicked in. This was the first time I remember thinking, "Now I know I can do this and so I'm going to push myself to see what I'm truly capable of."

I kept on going. I didn't change anything other than increasing the exercise volume a bit more. I got more and more focused. I did start occasionally going to a group fitness class called Inferno Hot Pilates. This was a class taught in a hot yoga studio. Some friends convinced me to try it and given how into fitness I was becoming, I figured what would be the harm in trying. I enjoyed it. These classes were essentially an hour-long sweat session of bodyweight movements in a humid 95-degree room filled with other sweaty people all trying to survive together. It was fun. Before I knew what had happened, it was already time for my next appointment.

3

December 20, 2021, 7:30am

I went in for my next appointment with Kaitie and we did another check-in. This time, my weight had dropped to 149 pounds. Now I had lost 9% of my body weight since July. Still, I could see no real body composition changes or muscle tone but clearly something was happening. After the nurse came to take more of my blood, I eagerly anticipated the results. Later that day I got them.

December 2021 Bloodwork Results

Measure	Result	Optimal Range
Total Cholesterol	227	140-200
Calculated LDL	122	0-129, <100 optimal
Cardiac Risk	5.3	0-5
Triglycerides	309	<150 optimal
HDL	43	>40 optimal
Non-HDL	184	---

Some of these numbers were a bit of a wake-up call. My total cholesterol actually went up. My triglycerides also went up. They didn't go up astronomically but after one precipitous drop between July and September, they were now creeping up again.

The good news was that my cardiac risk ratio had dropped a bit more and was now getting close to within the optimal range. The better news was that my HDL score, the good cholesterol, was finally high enough to be considered in the optimal range. That HDL number was the solace I took from this visit. I realized at that moment that progress as it relates to health is not necessarily linear. There are going to be ups and downs. These numbers certainly didn't deter me. In fact, they may have had the opposite effect. In some regards, I could argue that having some of those numbers tick up a bit was actually good for me because it was proof that there would be no quick fix and that I'd need to stay disciplined.

I couldn't understand why the numbers went up because I thought I had been doing all the right things. Back to work, I went. At this point, I had also started adding to the exercise equipment at home. I had started with just a Peloton bike but now I had added some dumbbells, a barbell with some weight plates, an adjustable bench, some resistance bands, and a TRX suspension trainer. I even had a small mirror leaning up against the wall that made me uncomfortable but allowed me to check my form from time to time. I always felt so weird seeing myself exercise. I was watching more and more YouTube videos and trying to put together actual workouts for myself that involved multiple different exercises. All of this equipment was in an unfinished part of our basement with some rubber puzzle-piece-style floor mats. I didn't really know what I was doing but I was having a great time doing it.

When my next appointment arrived — in March of 2022 — I had gotten more and more comfortable and confident with what

I was doing for my health. At this point, I was starting to see changes in my body that looked like a sliver of muscle definition. Mr. Olympia competition, here I come. I got my blood work at the March appointment and my total cholesterol went up a little from 227 in December to 235 in March as well as my cardiac risk going up a bit again to 5.7 in March from 5.3 in December. 5.7 was lower than where it was in July of 2021 but a tenth of a point higher than it was in September of 2021. My HDL had dropped a bit this time down to 41 so still in the optimal range. My triglycerides had dropped back down to 267 — down from 309 in December. I was a bloodwork yo-yo. I suppose this is what happens as you try to figure out how to hack your biology. Certainly, everything was better than it had been in July of 2021 but there was still plenty of figuring-out to do.

This went on for a while. In July of 2022, a year later, my triglycerides dropped to 236, their lowest yet. By January of 2023, those triglycerides were down to 137. Jackpot. They were finally in the optimal range. Also in January of 2023, my cardiac risk had dropped below 5 down to 4.4 which was now also in the optimal range. HDL had gone up to 50, well into the optimal range now. Things were going really well but there was no way I was stopping now. I was now trying to be the healthiest I'd ever been and to get myself into the best shape of my life.

While my triglycerides were dropping and my HDL was climbing, something else was happening beneath the surface. Each improvement in my numbers corresponded with a small boost in confidence — not just about my health, but about my capacity for change. I was discovering that transformation isn't compartmentalized; when you prove to yourself you can change one thing, you start questioning what else might be possible. The numbers were just the first layer of evidence that change was possible.

4

March, 2023

This is when a fairly significant moment in this journey happened. The blood work told one story of progress — measurable, quantifiable changes in my health. But there was another story developing in parallel. While the numbers were improving incrementally, I was starting to realize that my DIY approach to fitness might have limitations. Just as the blood tests provided objective data about my health, I needed objective expertise about my fitness approach. That's when I saw the Facebook post from an acquaintance of mine who was changing careers to follow a life-long passion of hers to become a personal trainer. I sent a message congratulating her for the career change and then half-jokingly asked her when she was going to put me on a program. We exchanged a few messages back and forth a bit and ended up on a phone call where all of a sudden I was explaining my whole situation to her. I ended up deciding to be her first client.

Her business model involved coming to clients' houses and working with them there, using their own equipment, to develop a workout schedule and a variety of different workout routines that they could do on their own. The plan was for her to come once a week initially and then once every other week to help me through one of the workouts. This, it turned out, was a revelation. Now I had someone who knew what they were doing putting together an actual plan for me rather than me just doing whatever I felt would work. What I didn't know right then but learned quickly is that I actually had grossly underestimated how important it is to actually know what you're doing; particularly if you want to achieve progress.

The workouts were way more challenging. I didn't have to think. I would go to my basement and look at the printed-out routine she sent me that was taped to the foundation wall and just do that. I loved it. I worked with her for 3 months. She gave me a variety of routines and pushed me to push myself. She was great. Through working with her I learned so much about different kinds of exercises including why it was important to sequence your workouts and to have proper rest time and how to lift with proper form. I learned that if you do too much cardio before you do your strength training, your body will be too tired to lift the weight you need to lift in order to be the most effective.

It really should have been more obvious: of course, a person with professional training would know better than I would. Of course, the progress I would make — physically and psychologically — would be better once I was doing things that were actually effective and well-programmed.

5

After 3 months of working out with her, June had rolled around and the summer was upon us. My family's schedule in the summer is a little fluid so I decided that I would take a break from the training visits but I would certainly not take a break from training. I was really loving it. At our last appointment, she and I discussed how it would have been fun to do proper before and after progress photos. It would have been something I could have to memorialize my progress so far and something she could use on her personal training social media. Yes indeed. A win-win situation for both of us. You see these all the time. It makes perfect sense. I had never taken a progress photo although now is probably the right time to tell you that since working with her, I had started to see significant body composition changes. I had real muscle definition now. The difference in progress between working on my own with a routine that I had *designed* by myself versus working with a personal trainer with a routine designed by someone who knew what they were doing was startling. I was easily in the best shape of my life at that point. Oh well. Maybe next time I have terrible cholesterol and am really out of shape I'll do a better job of proactively getting a photo for the next before.

She suggested we could still do it. I asked if she had a time machine because I wasn't sure how we would get a proper before photo. She told me I could use any photo I had of myself from before we started working out together. Any photo that showed what my body looked like in any way. I asked her what would be good for an after-photo. I think I had an idea in my head but immediately started to feel a sense of dread. She suggested, like what you see on TV commercials and social media all the time: shirtless and flexing. I think I blacked out. To be clear, she absolutely did nothing wrong and didn't ask for anything inappropriate. I simply had never done anything like that. I had exactly zero pictures of me shirtless — as a matter of fact — I don't think I had ever seen a picture of me shirtless other than when I was a baby or little kid. I asked her if I could think about it for a bit and get back to her. She said absolutely. She really is incredible and if you're in the Boston area and need a trainer, get in touch with me because I highly recommend her. She was so supportive the entire time.

I asked if I could blur my face and remain anonymous in the photos. While I couldn't articulate why this felt necessary, it seemed like the only way forward. She was supportive, as always.

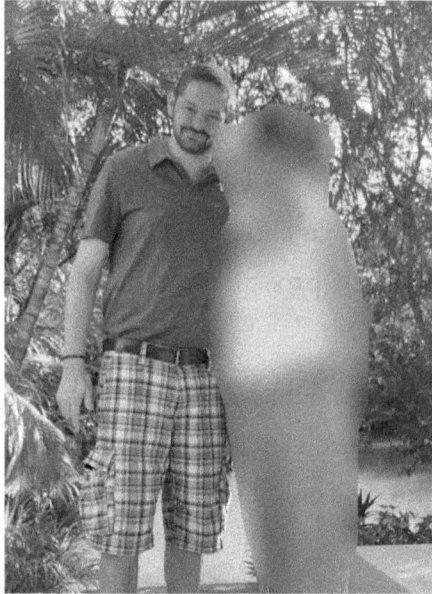

Similar to the "before" photo I sent her but my face was also blurred

I decided to do it. Before I got to really introspecting on why I was so nervous about taking an *after* photo and why I found it necessary to blur my face out of it and be anonymous, I had to figure out how to take the photo. In one of the more awkward moments of my life to date, I propped up my phone and took a few photos of myself, shirtless and flexing. By the way, flexing

— it turns out — is a skill I do not possess. Everything about it felt awkward. I took a few photos and then asked my wife to help me objectively pick which one I should use. We decided on one of them and I proceeded to blur my face out of it.

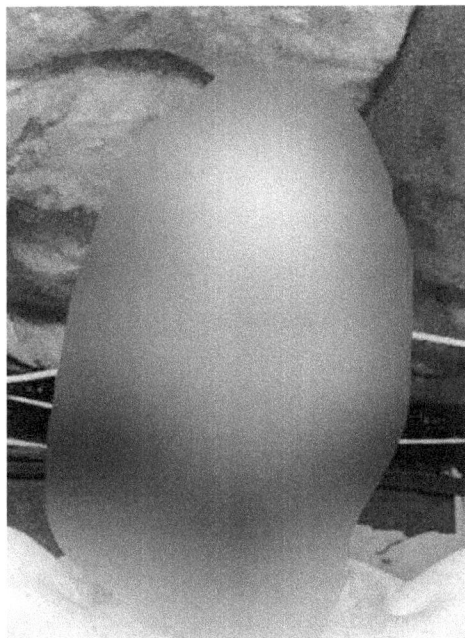

Here is the top of the photo that I ultimately sent to my trainer which she subsequently posted on social media. I intentionally zoomed in here to just show you the blurred part. This is the beginning of the moment that I alluded to at the beginning of this chapter. This was the moment when I started to explore my larger psychological history.

Again: why was I so nervous about this photo? What was I nervous about? Why did I decide to do it but with a blurred face? Why was it important to me to not have my name attached? These are all the questions I started to ask myself and what I will try to explore here. To be honest, it makes me very uncomfortable. As I've thought about how to write this chapter I have struggled — in a very meta way — with the very same thing that caused me to want to blur my face in the first place. This whole book is about self-discovery and transformation. There is a literal piece of evidence that I COULD share: the actual photo; all of it. You would see the physical result of the work I've put in.

Let's start with one piece of objectivity: progress photos are helpful. When you see yourself every day it is really difficult to see progress. Waiting three, six, or 12 months to get the next blood test is not as easy as just looking in the mirror. Having a photo that you can store away and then compare with a newer photo later is quite useful.

That's all well and good. I realized that for me, progress photos came with something else that was less objective: shame. I felt embarrassed to take the photo. I didn't want anyone who saw it to know it was me. What was I so embarrassed about? At the time that the photo was taken, I was a 45-year-old man in pretty good physical condition using it to demonstrate, objectively, the result of hard work. If you do really well on a test in school, you bring home that test with the big circled $A+$ circled on it to show your parents because you're proud of what you accomplished. When your daughter gets her driver's license, you post on Facebook some ridiculous joke about making sure people stay off the sidewalks now or that squirrels better watch out but what you're really doing is expressing your pride for your child's achievement. When a football player scores a touchdown or a basketball player hits a 3-pointer or a tennis player aces a serve the player might look to the crowd with a fist in the air.

People will cheer for the accomplishment. Why is this any different? This photo embodies all the hard work I'd put in to get myself healthy. What would be the harm in expressing that pride publicly?

Well, what if people interpret it as me being vain? What if they interpret it as me showing off? What if the *wrong* people see it (whoever the *wrong* people are)? Now I found myself spending more time feeling anxious about the photo than I was feeling happy about the achievement. I found myself with visible muscle definition for the first time in my life at the age of 45. But as I sat down to write this book about health, and longevity, I had to ask myself: why is that muscle tone relevant? Are visible abs important? Are they evidence of health or just evidence that I achieved a certain body fat percentage? And why was I both proud of them and uncomfortable sharing a photo that showed them?

The visible changes in my body, while not the most important health markers, were evidence that my new habits were creating real change. You can't see cholesterol improvements in a photo, but you can see the physical results of the same behaviors that improved those numbers. This photo didn't show health directly — but did show consistency, commitment, and change. That is ultimately why I decided it was ok to even talk about this here but it still didn't answer a clearly deeper-seated issue.

You know that moment in the movie when you start seeing rapid flashbacks to represent a character starting to piece together all the evidence? In "The Usual Suspects," there's a great version of this with Chazz Palminteri's character — Dave Kujan

— as he is figuring out the identity of the antagonist, Kaiser Soze. Dave Kujan is sitting on the edge of a different character's desk. This character — Jeff Rabin, played by Dan Hedaya — is listening as Dave comments that Jeff's desk and office is a mess. Jeff says, "It all makes sense when you look at it right. You have to stand back from it." Dave Kujan chuckles a bit and stares at the messy bulletin board as the camera slowly starts pushing in toward his face. The music starts playing and his expression changes from smiling to contemplative to realization. The audience sees a rapid sequence of moments from the movie we've already seen. This time they are strung together with various voiceovers and revelations as the big plot twist is revealed.

Over the next weeks and months after the blurred photo moment, I had a similar personal experience — albeit less dramatic and without any Academy Awards.

"The greatest trick the devil ever pulled was convincing the world he didn't exist." — Kaiser Soze, The Usual Suspects

When I was in middle school, if you played something like basketball in gym class — and there were two teams — it was not uncommon for one team to be the *shirts* team and the other team to be *skins* — the team that would have to play without shirts on. I remember dreading and ultimately trying to position myself during the shirts/skins/shirts/skins headcount that the teacher would do to make sure I was on the *shirts* team. At the time, I didn't know why other than I just didn't want to be on *skins*.

As I mentioned earlier in the chapter, I was not aware of any shirtless photos of myself from after I was maybe four or five years old. How is that even possible? I've been on the beach with my family and with friends. I've been to swimming pools (although never loved swimming — also interesting). There is incredibly limited evidence of me in any of these places. How about pictures of me from the honeymoon my wife and I went on to a tropical resort in Mexico? Surely there would be something from then? Nothing.

When I was in college for my freshman year, I lived in a dormitory that had shared bathrooms on each floor. Regularly people who go use the bathroom and walk down the hall in their towels before and after they took showers. Not me. I brought a shirt with me to the bathroom so I could take it off right before I got in the shower and put it back on before I walked back to my room. I went to summer camp for many many years. My best friends in the world come from that experience. At summer camp people are typically at their least guarded because everyone is just living dirty at camp and it's typically pretty hot out. I imagine there are many of my best camp friends in the world who have never seen me shirtless. I measure my involvement at this particular camp in decades. It runs during the warmest part of the year. You live in cabins that aren't air-conditioned. I imagine that I have many friends — some of whom I'm very close with — who have never seen me shirtless.

Remember that Inferno Hot Pilates class I mentioned earlier? The room it took place in was large enough to hold somewhere between 30 and 40 people on yoga mats. It is dimly lit with a full-length wall-to-wall mirror on one side. Given the heat in the room, most people are wearing limited clothing. There are all different bodies in the room including men and women who are clearly very fit and others who are clearly not. There are even pregnant women. Most of the women are wearing some sort of sports bra situation and shorts. Most of the men are in shorts and no shirt. When I first started going I wore shorts and a loose-fitting yoga shirt. I remember feeling very self-conscious; not only because I figured everyone would be looking at me (ridiculous and ultimately unfounded), but also because I could see via the mirror that so many of these people were really good at the exercises in the class. At certain points of the class, the instructor gives the orders to do a forearm plank. For those unfamiliar, this is when you are face down as if you are about to do a pushup but instead, you just rest on your forearms and your toes so your body is parallel to the ground. You just hold the position for a while. Imagine being in a room that is humid and 95 degrees facing down with a loose-fitting shirt. My face would inevitably end up essentially staring into the neck hole of the shirt. This was lovely if you are into breathing in your own hot breath combined with sweat. At one point — a few classes into this for me — I decided enough was enough and took my shirt off. It was incredibly freeing physically. I decided that the risk of anyone judging me (wasn't actually happening) was not worth suffering in the heat through my outfit choice.

6

The moments kept piling up. While I had never put any of it together before and certainly never remembered really worrying about any of these moments other than trying to avoid being put into a circumstance that I thought might make me uncomfortable, there was clearly a pattern that I never recognized until the blurred photo.

Did I have deep-seated body image issues? I think the answer must be yes.

This — for me — is related to a lack of confidence that I dealt with when I was younger, in certain areas of my life. I have always been very confident in my professional skills. I feel like I am good at what I do for a living and I feel like other people think that too. I have always felt pretty good about my career and the way I have navigated that. Relationships, though, were a different story. I was never good at navigating relationships. I had no long-term girlfriends prior to meeting my now-wife. As a matter of fact, one of the things that drew me to her and ultimately acted as the catalyst for why I fell in love with her was that she made me feel more confident. She taught me that it was ok to be who I was. She was the first person who made me feel loved and desirable; from a relationship perspective. I had plenty of friends who were girls but that's usually where the relationship hit a plateau. In my mind, I am the original member of the friend zone — even if I didn't coin the phrase.

Are confidence and body image related? Of course they are. When we hear about people who struggle with their body image in society, we almost always hear about women. There have been surveys[12] on male body image that revealed between 20-40% of

---

[12] Eating Recovery Center's "Men Have Body Image Issues Too" - https://www.eatingrecoverycenter.com/resources/men-have-body-image-issues-too

men were unhappy with some aspects of their looks. People who struggle with their body image often reduce their social interactions, find ways to avoid intimate relationships, have a lower self-efficacy in dating situations, and deal with confidence silos (differing levels of confidence in different parts of their lives). This all seemed very relatable to me. Of course, because of how society defines a traditional "man" or "manly behavior" it is not surprising that many men don't want to discuss their body image concerns. The 20-40% statistic likely understates the reality. Men are less likely to report or discuss body image concerns due to societal expectations of masculinity. We're taught that caring about our appearance is vanity, that discussing insecurities is weakness, and that we should just 'man up' and deal with it. This creates a paradox where men simultaneously experience body image issues and feel shame about having those feelings in the first place. It's no wonder these issues often go unrecognized — we're culturally conditioned to ignore them, even within ourselves. What if it turns out that the confidence that I feel and show professionally is at least in part to compensate for the lack of confidence in other areas of my life?

Here is some good news: at the beginning of the book I encountered an acute problem with my health thanks to incredibly high cholesterol. Having that problem identified for me became the catalyst to start on a journey with a destination that I thought I knew. Through that process, I discovered — here — that there was likely an additional chronic problem. Once I had that realization I could start to address that too.

And then there was another big piece of evidence that — I think — was the beginning of starting to feel more resolved and at ease. I have a great friend who I met at the aforementioned summer camp. Her family doesn't live close to mine, so I don't get to see her very often. In August of 2021, she and her children were in town visiting her parents. They came over to our house for the afternoon to hang out at our pool. At some point during the visit, she wanted to take a picture. She asked one of her kids to take a picture of us. Here is that picture (with her face blurred out to protect her privacy):

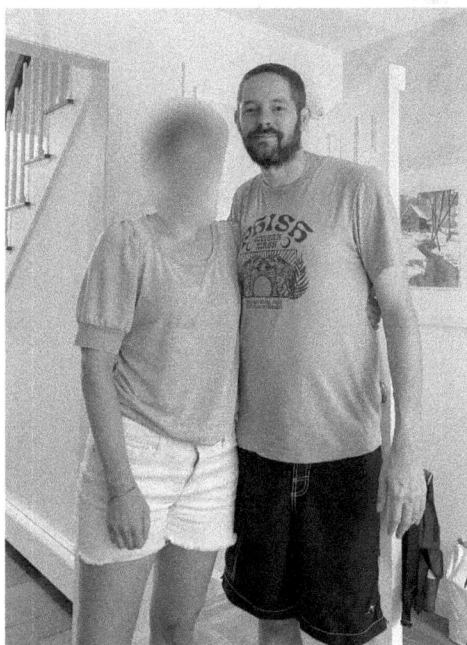

Here you can get a good sense of the true dadbod situation going on with me. At the time I didn't realize it. Remember, this was in August of 2021 and was less than a month after the original high cholesterol reveal. Now skip ahead to August of 2023; two years later. We saw each other again, this time on the last day of summer camp where we were both picking up our respective kids. Again, we decided to take a photo. Later that day she sent me a text message with the new photo (and I blurred her face again to protect her privacy). In it, I'm wearing a t-shirt that reads 'I am Kenough' — a bit of self-unaware humor about male body image that would have been unthinkable for me just a few years earlier:

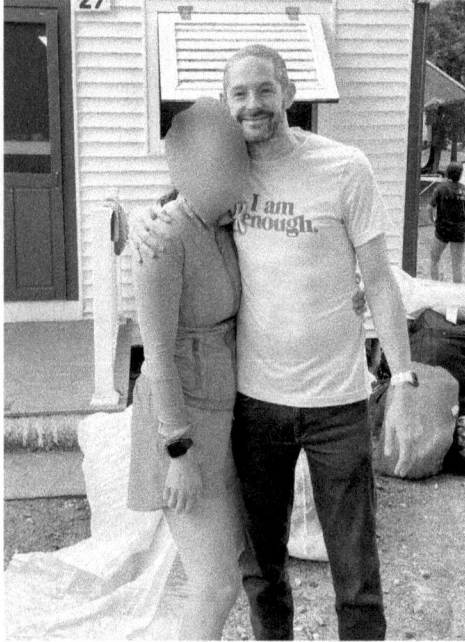

I am Kenough

I replied and mentioned that I could sort of see some abs through the shirt. She said she didn't want to say it before I did. She then sent me the photo from two years earlier. She said, "[I] definitely radiate more happiness now." I am choosing to share these photos and not the full blurred face and shirtless photo for a specific reason. These photos with my friend were organic, not designed to be staged like a progress photo, and captured something greater than the physical change. They happen to be both taken in the same position and show a good representation of progress for me in more ways than one.

My wife is my safe space and the person I trust the most and feel the most comfortable with. She had noticed a difference in my body composition throughout this process. She tells me the truth and has been a great objective validator for me. It's difficult to see changes in yourself. I looked to her for a little boost of confidence then and still do now.

When my friend sent me this new photo, it was the first time I felt like someone outside of my little bubble, who doesn't see me very often, had noticed and was recognizing the changes in me. I wasn't entirely sure how I felt about that at the time but we'll explore that soon. Look closer at these pictures, side by side:

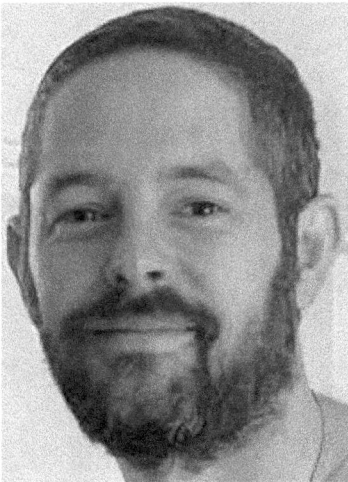

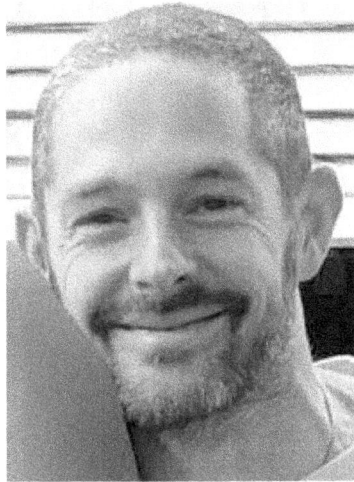

I thought I was on to something once I started to see the cholesterol numbers improve and I was. It turns out, however, that the real work hadn't revealed itself yet. Do you see it in those pictures? This isn't just about lowering cholesterol. This isn't about visible muscle definition. They are just evidence of a working process. I settled for being fine for a long time. The picture on the left was what I thought being fine meant. The picture on the right feels like it might be much closer to where I want to be.

Remember that topic I didn't see coming, the one I mentioned at the start? The one that took more time to figure out how to write about than any other part of this book? It wasn't really about the photos at all. The photos just finally made visible what had been there all along: decades of unacknowledged body image issues that had shaped my behaviors, my confidence, and my relationships. Like Kaiser Soze, these issues had been hiding in plain sight, convincing me they didn't exist. The greatest trick my body image issues ever pulled was convincing me I didn't have any.

But now I could see them. And once you can see something, you can begin to address it.

***

Something to think about...

What hidden barriers might be affecting your personal relationship with health or fitness?

CHAPTER SIX

BUILDING SOMETHING BETTER

1

What started as improving my cholesterol numbers evolved into building a healthier body. But somewhere along the way, I realized I was actually building something much more comprehensive: a better relationship with exercise, with my body, with food, and with myself.

If you look at a complete jigsaw puzzle — all put together — you see the whole picture and might not think too much about how many pieces make up the puzzle. Sometimes that puzzle has a smaller number of large pieces and sometimes it has a larger number of small pieces. As I was growing up, I was only aware of the "complete" puzzle and had no real understanding of the pieces that made it up. As I've gone through this journey, my understanding of the make-up of the puzzle has evolved. In the beginning, the one big piece of the puzzle was to lower my bad cholesterol. In the process of figuring out how to do that, I learned that physical activity — exercise — was a piece of the puzzle I had to get familiar with. While learning about that, I discovered a new piece of the puzzle: my sense of confidence and body image complexities. As this book goes on, I will continue to explore both of those topics but first, there's another big piece of the puzzle that I have had to learn about: nutrition.

While exercise was teaching me about physical capability, nutrition was teaching me something equally valuable: the power of intentional choices. Every meal became an opportunity to build something better, though it would take time to understand exactly what that meant.

I've discussed intermittent fasting — a form of restrictive dieting — and why my doctor thought it would be beneficial for me. For the purposes of setting context, I think it is important to go over some of the most common types of dieting, at least at high levels. In chapter 9 I'll explore the concept of "quick-fix" solutions but here, let's go over some of the basics. Most commonly, people are interested in this diet or that diet with the intention of losing weight. As I've established earlier, that was not the goal for me. That being said, intermittent fasting is one mechanism people have tried in order to lose weight. In Chapter 4 I talked about the most basic weight loss concept: consume more calories than you burn and you will gain weight while burning more calories than you consume will cause you to lose weight. For many people, I think they believe that intermittent fasting is a framework that will force them to consume fewer calories than they otherwise would have if they weren't restricting their food intake to a time window.

This doesn't always work. One of the common pitfalls for people trying intermittent fasting is that they feel like they can eat whatever they want in their time window. In that case, they might actually be consuming more calories than they would have if they spaced out their eating over the course of the day. Because I was doing the 16:8 version of intermittent fasting — eating in an eight-hour window and fast for 16 hours — I was full most of the time and simply couldn't overeat. My appetite couldn't handle it. I lost too much weight until I figured out the right mix of nutrition — in the form of what I was actually eating — and how to space out my meals in the window.

The interesting thing about intermittent fasting was that it forced me to think about food differently. It wasn't just about when to eat anymore — it was about making conscious decisions about what to eat. This was my first real step toward understanding nutrition as a tool for building rather than just a way to avoid hunger.

2

There are other forms of intermittent fasting as well. The 16:8 method is probably the most common and worked really well for me. Much of that 16 hours of fasting happened while I was sleeping. There is also an alternative day-fasting approach. With this approach, someone will eat relatively normally for one day, and on the next day they will either completely fast or consume a low number of calories. This can be beneficial because on the fast days, your body has much more time to clean itself up (autophagy) but can be really challenging if you're the type of person who ever socializes with other people. It is a pretty aggressive approach.

Yes, another intermittent fasting style is the 5:2 approach. This is when you eat normally for five days a week and then for the other two you heavily restrict your caloric intake. This gives you a bit more flexibility but the change to lower calories after five days of normal eating can be challenging. When I started my 16:8 intermittent fasting, it took my body a few days to adjust to the new eating schedule but that schedule was the same every day. In the 5:2 approach, your body is essentially re-training itself every week.

Of course, there are other types of diets including all the brand-name diets. It seems to be pretty common for people to associate the word "diet" with the concept of losing weight but I prefer to think of it using its primary definition: food and drink regularly provided or consumed[13].

Whatever the reason is for the choice you make about how you eat and what you eat, I encourage you to be intentional and acknowledge that not every mechanism works for every person. Even if you were exactly the same person as me with exactly the same cholesterol issues and the exact same metabolism and you were my age and my height and my weight, 16:8 intermittent fasting might not be right for you. You should definitely talk with

---

[13] Merriam-Webster definition of the word diet: https://www.merriam-webster.com/dictionary/diet

your doctor before trying any of these methods to make sure it's healthy for you.

Intermittent fasting was just the framework for the time-restricted food intake. The bigger aspect of this for me — as it relates to the nutrition piece of my puzzle — was actually *what* I ate more than *when* I ate it. Let's talk about that.

3

In Chapter 4 I talked a bit about the main macronutrients: protein, carbohydrates, and fats. Understanding how these all work — and what their values are — as they relate to your goals is important and then subsequently, how you actually measure them. To recap a bit on the value of those macros: protein is essential for muscle maintenance and immune function. It is also satiating and will fill you up. This is good if you're trying to reduce the number of calories you are taking in. I pay attention to my protein intake more than any other macro. Carbohydrates provide fiber which attaches to cholesterol and removes it from your body. Soluble (the good) fiber can help reduce LDL (the bad) cholesterol. Healthy fats will help raise HDL (the good) cholesterol. Unhealthy fats, like what you'd see referred to as trans fats or saturated fats can raise your LDL cholesterol. They all work together. Fiber from carbohydrates helps to remove cholesterol. Healthy fats help move and balance cholesterol levels, and protein supports overall metabolic health.

Understanding these numbers was empowering. Instead of just following rules, I was learning to make informed choices. It's like learning the language of your body — suddenly you can have real conversations instead of just nodding along.

Tracking these macros — and calories in general — has been really helpful for me but comes with risks. It can be a bit of a double-edged sword. There are plenty of apps that you can use for this type of tracking. Many of the apps allow you to scan barcodes or enter specific food items. They have a library of foods with nutritional information that will keep running tallies during the day of the macros and calories. At least at the beginning of my journey, this was a really helpful tool for me to gauge how much of each thing I was eating. Most of these types of apps also let you set goals, have recipes, and offer comprehensive nutritional insights. That is the good edge of the sword. The other edge is tricky, particularly if you have obsessive-compulsive tendencies like me.

Even though I don't consider myself a foodie, I do like to enjoy the food I'm eating. In a similar way to the exercise part of my life I was learning, I have always tried to be cognizant of getting obsessive. Like most adults, I have lots of things going on in my life and responsibilities to attend to in addition to my health. Getting laser-focused on calorie tracking or obsessive about making sure I have exactly the right amount of carbs or precisely the right amount of protein is a slippery slope.

It ultimately became about a mindset for me. Whatever my goals were, are, or will be revolve around milestones like lowering my cholesterol or getting in shape or making better food choices. None of the milestones have specific timeframes. That is the key for me. Applying an arbitrary timeframe to the goals yields manufactured stress. Once that happens, I could see myself getting anxious if I happened to have a day when I didn't hit one of the macro goals. That anxiety could snowball into a bigger problem the next day. It turns out that not every day is perfect and that's ok. The moment I resolved to do the best I could while still making sure I enjoyed my day-to-day life and that I could balance the priority of getting healthier with the other priorities in my life, the stress melted away. Not having that stress contributes to the enjoyment factor for the rest of the process and that makes it more likely that I'll achieve the daily goals which in turn makes it more likely that I'll achieve the longer-term goals.

So I found a way to track my nutritional intake without increasing my stress levels. I've tried a few different apps for this over the years and will not include any sort of recommendation here. You should look around at the different types of apps and figure out what works for you; which is exactly how every other topic in this book should be.

Back to protein. This was the macronutrient that I was the most interested in. You just won't build muscle if you don't consume enough protein. The general rule of thumb for protein intake — if you're looking to build muscle — is 1.0 to 1.2 grams of protein per pound of your body weight. I was hovering between 150 and 155 pounds at the time I started paying attention to macros — and protein specifically. That means that I was aiming for anywhere between 150 and 190 (rounding up) grams of protein per day. Protein is very filling. Here is a rough example of what that actually might look like:

A filet mignon steak might be around six to 10 ounces. On the low end that might be around 40 to 45 grams of protein. That same filet is probably under 400 calories. I'd have to have four of those per day in order to hit the protein goals. Those four filets would be 1600 calories for the day and 180 grams of protein; roughly. Even at 1600 calories — which would be pretty low for me — I would feel very full. Compare that with, let's say, a serving of Chips Ahoy chocolate chip cookies. A single serving is made up of three cookies and is 160 calories and one gram of protein. So eight Chips Ahoy cookies are roughly the same amount of calories as a 6oz filet mignon. Those 8 cookies will get you about 2 grams of protein vs the 40+ you'd get from the filet. Also, I'd be willing to bet that after you had those cookies you'd be hungry again pretty quickly, unlike how you feel after you eat a filet.

Unnaturally sugary foods like cookies cause your blood glucose levels to spike, similar to what was happening to me when I drank all that Coca-Cola. When that spike happens your pancreas kicks into high gear and releases a lot of insulin. The insulin is charged with getting that sugar out of your bloodstream but because of how quickly the spike happened, the insulin is essentially acting aggressively and can leave your blood sugar levels even lower than where they were before you ate the cookies. Your body overcompensates. This makes you even hungrier. This is what the Chips Ahoy people want. Now I need to go buy more cookies.

I do love chocolate chip cookies though. Just for fun, if I wanted to get 180g of protein just from Chips Ahoy chocolate chip cookies I would have to eat over 500 cookies a day. You know, that doesn't sound all that bad. This kind of knowledge changed how I viewed food choices. It wasn't about *good* or *bad* foods anymore — it was about understanding what different choices would do for my goals. The cookies didn't become forbidden; they just became a choice I could make with full awareness.

The point here is that protein is satiating — it fills you up — and I tried to prioritize that over other foods. Take the four filets I'd have to eat in a day to get 180 grams of protein and now add another layer of complexity: I was intermittent fasting so I was only eating from noon through 8 pm. With proper spacing, I'd have to eat a full 6oz filet mignon at noon then again at around 2:15 pm then again around 4:45 pm, and then again around 7:15 pm. There's no way that would happen. Of course, I'm being ridiculous but hopefully, the point is clear: trying to consume a lot of other protein because it's necessary to build muscle knowing that it's very filling while also intermittent fasting is really challenging. This is likely why you don't see a lot of bodybuilders who do intermittent fasting and why I am not a bodybuilder (that's the only reason).

Intermittent fasting and high protein intake have competing interests. This is why it's so important to really understand what your goals are and what systems work for you. It took me quite a while to figure out the combination of foods that I could eat (and enjoyed eating) that would give me the amount of protein I was looking for but not be so filling that I was walking around like a stuffed pig all day. I introduced high-protein yogurt and replaced sugary snacks with protein shakes so that everything I was eating had at least some measurable protein value. This took me quite a while to figure out how to do it properly.

There's another wrinkle to consider. According to the Federal Drug Administration of the United States (FDA):

> Class II nutrients are vitamins, minerals, protein, total carbohydrate, dietary fiber, other carbohydrate, polyunsaturated and monounsaturated fat, or potassium that occur naturally in a food product. Class II nutrients must be present at 80% or more of the value declared on the label.[14]

That means there's a good chance that the actual amount of protein (or other macros) you get might not be what you see on the label. If the cup of yogurt says 20g of protein it might actually be 16g. The good news is that you don't have to lick the cup dry in order to get whatever the full amount is. Those numbers typically account for the reasonable consumable portion contained within the packaging. It's quite a bit easier to measure protein in whole natural foods like chicken or turkey or steak or salmon but in pre-packaged foods like the protein shakes I drink or the yogurt, there's a built-in margin for error. To cover for that potential short-fall, I typically aim for closer to 200g of protein per day. As my understanding of nutrition grew, so did my confidence in making food choices. What started as a confusing maze of numbers and percentages became a toolkit for building the body — and the health — I wanted.

---

[14] FDA on Nutritional Labels: https://www.fda.gov/regulatory-information/search-fda-guidance-documents/guidance-industry-guide-developing-and-using-data-bases-nutrition-labeling

4

Looking back, I realize nutrition wasn't just another piece of the puzzle — it was the mortar that held other pieces together. Better nutrition supported better workouts, which built more confidence and encouraged better food choices. Each element strengthened the others.

This is my advice: do the best that you can. I don't have time in my life to weigh everything or track everything or look everything up. I just guess — in an educated way. I try to eat things that are a bit better for me rather than the things that I know are a bit worse for me. These are deliberate choices that I chose to make and you can do the same. If you were eating the way I was and you want to get healthier, these are the types of things you have to choose to do. This doesn't mean it can't be fun or that you can't enjoy food. It doesn't mean you have to get it right every day. Sometimes I like partaking in a piece of chocolate cake. I don't regret it. Allowing myself the chocolate cake makes me feel good in the moment because there's no timeline for the goal. Live your life.

***

Something to think about...

When was the last time you ate your favorite dessert?

PART THREE

PHYSICAL EVIDENCE

CHAPTER SEVEN

THE EXPECTATION CHASM

1

I thought it would be simple: eat better, move more, get healthy. Like following a recipe or assembling a desk-hutch-couch combo unit from Ikea — just follow the instructions and voila! We've been conditioned to expect to see our desired outcome immediately. I'll refer to this as the *Primification Phenomenon*. When I shop for anything using Amazon's Prime service, I'm optimizing for what will get to me fastest. If there is something that's rated five stars but won't arrive until tomorrow and something that's rated four stars but will arrive sometime today between 10 am and 2 pm, I'm picking the latter. Four stars is good enough and I just can't wait until tomorrow.

This urgency to get what I want — or even what I need — right now can lead to a compromise in quality. There's also the disappointment I feel when the thing I need — whatever it is — has no option of arriving quickly. This is of course quite a shift from the days of sending in the form you'd get from the mail-order catalog and having to wait three to six months for whatever it is you ordered. I need it now.

Just like expecting same-day delivery for every purchase, I found myself wanting same-week results for every workout. Surely if I did fifty crunches today, I'd see abs tomorrow. If I ate one healthy meal, shouldn't my cholesterol drop in some measurable way? This desire for instant transformation isn't just impatience — it's become our default setting. My instinct is to try and attain the goals as quickly as possible and no matter how quickly that ends up being, it won't be quick enough. I'm not entirely sure who, if anyone, is to blame for this and perhaps that's not even important. The expectations that we often set for ourselves — including how long it will take to get to whatever outcome it is that we're looking for — are usually unrealistic.

2

In Chapter 9 I'll discuss why I think the distance between expectation and reality as it relates to health and fitness is so vast. When I'm shopping for toilet paper or those revolutionary new stackable coffee mugs, if I have to wait a few extra days it's disappointing but ultimately not that big a deal. With health and fitness — the latter more so — there are risks; potentially significant ones. Let's make up a scenario; albeit one that is not that far-fetched for many people.

Let's say you decide to run a local 5k charity race in two weeks. Your goal: run a mile in under 10 minutes, projecting a 30-minute 5k finish. You haven't run since high school PE class 25+ years ago, but how hard could it be?

You tell yourself that this is going to go great and not only that, you think maybe you'll just keep training after and be ready for the marathon that's happening in a few months. You'll just start doing some light jogging each day for a few days to "warm up." After a few days you're feeling pretty good about yourself because you haven't died yet. You're even doing some stretching because you know that's the right thing to do. A few days in and you decide that you're ready to try to run a timed mile. You start your run and about a quarter of a mile in you take a break to walk for a bit because it's been a long time since you've run any sort of distance and it turns out you can't breathe. You finish the mile with a combination of walking and jogging but you definitely sprint the final 100 feet just in case anyone is watching. You check and see that it took you 16 minutes.

Now, with just over a week to go, you figure you'll just speed up a bit each time. You figure that if you can get it down to a 12-minute mile prior to race day, you'll get the last two minutes via adrenaline like you hear about from people who run marathons. You quickly realize on the next day of training that you're losing your breath much faster, your feet are starting to hurt pretty quickly, and your ankles are really sore after each run. You still push yourself for a few days because you're determined to succeed. You come home and your wife asks why you're limping. You didn't even notice. You spend the rest of the day with your foot elevated because your ankle has swelled up. Also, you have developed some blisters.

You're now a few days away from the race and are annoyed — but not dissuaded — because you had to skip a few days of running due to the blisters but you're ok with it because your ankle has been bothering you in a sort of persistent way so you figured the rest now would allow you to get back to running soon enough. You decide — to your credit — that you're still going to keep trying. The day before the race you'll just walk a few miles because at least that's something. and your blisters and ankle could use the break. You don't mind because tomorrow's the 5k and who cares how you feel after that?

The day of the race arrives and you feel ready to go. You've worked hard and tell yourself that everyone has bumps and bruises. The race starts and you power through the first mile. It takes you about 14 minutes. Your feet are killing you and you will definitely need some ice for that ankle later. You spend most of the second mile walking and then get back to some light jogging for the third mile because you want to finish strong. You finish the race. You're proud of yourself — as you should be — but deep down you're also disappointed because your race time was 46 minutes.

You tell yourself that maybe the 10-minute mile goal in two weeks was a bit too ambitious. If the goal had simply been to finish the race without unrealistic expectations, you might have felt better about it all and avoided the sprained ankle and infected blisters.

If the expectations are not realistic when it comes to fitness you are either risk hurting yourself to try and meet them, disappointing yourself when you don't meet them, or both. If we can be patient and wait for the extra day or two to get the revolutionary stackable coffee mugs then we can be patient while we work to achieve whatever the fitness goal is.

This isn't just about running. Whether it's strength training, weight loss, or cholesterol improvement, unrealistic expectations don't just disappoint us — they can actively harm us. Understanding this gap between expectation and reality isn't about lowering our goals — it's about setting ourselves up for actual success.

3

Let's look at another scenario. Your doctor tells you your cholesterol is high (sound familiar?) or maybe you've decided you want to lose 20 pounds before summer. You decide you're going to completely transform your eating habits starting Monday. You clear out your pantry of anything processed, spend $300 at Whole Foods on Sunday, and plan to meal prep for the week. You've watched some health influencers on social media do this — it looks simple enough. Just lean protein, whole grains, and vegetables six times a day. You'll get all your containers ready on Sunday night.

Monday goes great. Your food doesn't look as good as food in the video you saw from this one influencer but it tastes pretty good and you think this will be fine to eat every day. By Wednesday, you've started to question if this is going to work because you're already getting bored of having the same meals every day. You decide it's ok to just take one meal off and then feel guilty about the $15 salad you bought at lunch instead of eating what you prepped. Because you only had a salad for lunch and are really hungry, you spend the afternoon thinking about the food you "can't" have. You're wondering why you don't feel amazing yet. You're also getting anxious about the weekend because you're supposed to go out with some a friend for their birthday dinner. There will definitely be some chocolate cake. You tell yourself it's ok because you'll just start next Monday.

The cycle of restrictive eating and guilt isn't just unsustainable — it creates a psychological burden that makes the whole process harder. What if, instead of expecting complete dietary transformation overnight, you took some baby steps? What if you told yourself you're going to replace one sugar snack per day with a piece of fruit and you're going to cut out soda? The longer-term goal is still to reduce your cholesterol or to lose 20 pounds but you aren't trying to do it all at once in a way that you won't be able to keep up with.

4

I know this cycle because I've lived it. That Sunday night feeling of virtue as you portion out identical meals into identical containers. The Wednesday realization that you're already sick of chicken and broccoli. The mental gymnastics of trying to convince yourself that this is a "lifestyle change" while simultaneously counting the days until you can go back to eating "normal" food again.

What I didn't understand then was that this wasn't just about food — it was about expecting instant transformation, both physical and mental. I thought that if I could just follow the perfect plan perfectly, everything would fall into place perfectly. Perfection, it turns out, is the enemy of progress.

A child needs time to develop language skills or learn to walk and we allow that grace. We don't expect them to reconcile their QuickBooks file within weeks of being born. It shouldn't be unreasonable to expect that our bodies and minds need appropriate time to adapt to new physical demands and lifestyle changes before we expect to achieve the desired outcome. Trying to rush this natural progression often leads to setbacks or injury.

There's an article on Psychology Today by Andrea Bonoir, Ph.D. called "7 New Year's Resolutions Bound to Fail[15]." Two of the resolutions that are bound to fail are joining a gym and eating healthier. According to Dr. Bonoir on joining a gym:

> We all know that gym memberships skyrocket after the holidays, even if the vast majority of those new exercisers clear out by Valentine's Day. Instead, you need a much better behavioral yardstick, so that you can build consistency in the habit and even reward yourself when you measure up. In fact, why give your money to the gym at all if it's not particularly convenient or realistic? Start smaller with what you've got. "Take the stairs to my office on Friday," or "Park in that way-off spot on Monday," will jumpstart far more tangible progress. And if you choose a daily goal, keep it small-- and know that

---

[15] 7 New Year's Resolutions Bound to Fail by Andrea Bonoir, Ph.D. - https://www.psychologytoday.com/us/blog/friendship-20/201412/7-new-years-resolutions-bound-to-fail

doing it for two or three weeks straight will help the habit solidify.

And on eating healthier:

> Vagueness, once again, is the downfall of this resolution. "Eat Healthier" also implies an overly aspirational rehaul of the type of person you are: after all, how we eat is a pretty big part of our being. Stay yourself, but just with a few small actions. How about starting to do Meatless Mondays? Or replacing the pasta you make most often with whole wheat? Or learning how to cook one new healthy meal by the 15th of each month? These changes allow for you to pat yourself on the back as you go, and they significantly reduce the possibility that you'll go "all-or-none" and feel like you've "failed" before the holiday decorations even come down.

Sports psychology research offers interesting insights. Studies show that athletes who focus on "process goals" (consistent small improvements) rather than "outcome goals" (dramatic quick results) not only perform better but also maintain their progress longer[16]. The science is clear: sustainable change requires patience, not just determination.

Understanding the gap between expectation and reality isn't about lowering our goals — it's about approaching them intelligently. In my case, once I stopped expecting overnight transformation and started focusing on consistent small

---

[16] From Weinberg and Gould in "Foundations of Sports and Exercise Psychology: https://www.trine.edu/academics/centers/center-for-sports-studies/blog/2023/the_relationship_between_self-confidence_and_performance.aspx#:~:text=Research%20and%20interviews%20with%20both,(Weinberg%20%26%20Gould%202019).

improvements, something interesting happened. The real, lasting change began to take shape.

But that's getting ahead of the story. First, let me show you what actual progress looked like — not the highlight reel version, but the messy, non-linear reality that eventually led to lasting change.

***

Something to think about...

Where are your expectations about health and fitness coming from? Are they serving you?

CHAPTER EIGHT

LIVING PROOF

1

Real progress doesn't follow a schedule. It doesn't arrive in an Amazon Prime box or show up on demand. My actual journey of transformation looked nothing like I expected — it was messier, slower, and ultimately more meaningful than any highlight reel or quick-fix solution could capture. While Chapter 7 showed what we often expect from change, let me show you what change actually looked like for me when I gave it the time and space to happen naturally.

The problem I was originally facing had no obvious way to define a realistic timeline. I just assumed I'd take care of "it" quickly. After I took action and made changes to the way I was living my life I saw my triglycerides drop from 1036 in July of 2021 down to 282 in September of 2021. That 73% drop gave me a false sense of confidence and why wouldn't it have? At that moment in time, it was basically proof that what I had changed *worked* and that was all there was to it. Three months later when the triglycerides went back up to 309 — a 9.5% increase — I was confused. The things I had changed in July were the same things I was doing that allowed for the 73% drop. How could those things now have allowed a 9.5% increase? As I introduced in Chapter 5, there were other things that I hadn't even discovered yet that would also require work and would warrant some progress. When I started the journey I was looking to make progress in one area. Through the journey I ended up figuring out that I was making progress in three, but the progress didn't meet my expectations until I learned enough — or at least more — about how my body and mind worked and then ultimately adjusted my expectations.

The reality of progress starts with one basic premise: it is different for everyone and defined by you. The moment you let someone else do that for you is the same moment you're setting yourself to be disappointed. This isn't to say that you can't or shouldn't get help or guidance from people who know more about how to achieve your goals but ultimately, you're the driver. Small and attainable goals — more about outputs than about outcomes — will make it much more likely that you'll actually stick with whatever plan you take on. I also believe that the goals should take the form of *strongly opinionated but loosely held*. By this, I mean that you should be committed to your goals and also allow yourself to be flexible as you go on your journey. I learned things along the way that I didn't have prior knowledge of that caused me to change the goals. That's a pivot; not a failure.

2

So let's talk about progress. Progress, for me, is tracked in different ways — some tangible and others less so — depending on the goals. Let's talk about physical progress first. If your goal is to lose 10 pounds the sort of obvious way to measure your progress would be to step on a scale. The thing to watch out for, though, is the "are we there yet" approach. Some people weigh themselves every day because their plan is to adjust their eating strategy each day depending on what the scale says. A weight-loss goal — like any other goal — is likely to be a non-linear rollercoaster. Some days you'll go up and other days you'll go down. Maybe you had a particularly stressful day and ate a lot. Maybe you had a fun dinner with friends. Maybe it was Thanksgiving and you ate dinner at 3:00 pm and that threw off your whole day. Maybe you had a busy day at work and missed lunch entirely. We have busy lives with more things to do than we have time for. Give yourself a little grace. Weighing yourself every day is almost certainly more likely to be a maddening exercise than a useful one. There's no progress that happens overnight so there's no reason to check your weight every day. I weigh myself every three or four weeks (but I'm not doing it for my weight — maybe that's confusing). I try to do it first thing in the morning before I've eaten anything to get the purest measurement and for consistency. Consistency is really important.

I don't weigh myself because I care about my weight. If you remember from earlier in the book, I wasn't trying to lose weight. I was trying to lower my cholesterol and there isn't a scale for that. It wasn't until I really started working out that I started to step on the scale but like I said, that wasn't about weight. That was about a metric that I think is even more important than weight; particularly if you have a goal of building muscle: body fat percentage.

3

Let's talk about body fat percentage.

When I first started tracking body fat, I thought my bathroom scale told me everything I needed to know. As I dug deeper into understanding my progress, I discovered a whole world of measurement methods. Each had its own strengths and limitations.

Body fat percentage is the amount of fat in your body compared to everything else including muscles, bones, organs, and water. For example, if you weighed 155 pounds and had a body fat percentage of 25%, that would mean that almost 39 pounds of your 155 would be fat and around 116 pounds of lean mass (muscles, bones, organs, etc). What kind of fat you have and where it's stored matters. Visceral fat — like I talked about in chapter 1 — is bad for you. It's the stubborn stuff that surrounds your organs and makes it harder for them to do their jobs. It also increases your inflammation. Generally speaking, the less muscle you have the lower your metabolic rate will be. You will have reduced strength and your body will have a reduced ability to regulate sugar. Your bones and joints will have less support. While some fat is definitely good, the preference would be to have subcutaneous fat (the outer blanket you can pinch) rather than visceral fat.

Now let's say — as another example — that you weighed the same 155 pounds but were 13% body fat. In that case, you would have 20 pounds of fat and 135 pounds of lean mass. Same exact weight but 19 fewer pounds of you are fat because those 19 pounds are lean mass. They are helping to support your bones and joints. They are helping your body work more efficiently. This is why weight, to me, is much less important. Relatively speaking, my weight hasn't changed all that much but my body fat percentage has changed drastically. This is generally referred to as your body composition. Since I figured out how to actually do intermittent fasting my weight has essentially stayed the same for two years. If I used weight as a way to gauge progress, I'd have concluded that I made none. The composition of my body changed though; my body fat percentage.

You can put away the vanity for a minute and just think objectively. Body fat varies based on your sex. Women's and men's bodies need and present body fat differently. For example, men who are over 30% body fat are considered obese — regardless of their actual weight. 25-29% is an above-average body fat percentage. 18-24% is considered to be healthy for a man. 14-17% is where someone who is pretty fit might fall. In this range, you might see muscle definition and maybe some of those visible abs. 6-13% is generally where athletes or really fit people land. There are almost definitely visible abs at this point and the muscle definition is really clear. Below 6% is generally not sustainable or healthy. There are some bodybuilders who get down that low for a competition or show but it's not a place where anyone would or should stay for long.

For women, the numbers are different. We have different bodies with different needs so that isn't a surprise. For women, a percentage over 37% is considered obese. 32-36% is an above-average percentage of body fat for women. 25-31% is the average to healthy range. 21-24% is the fit range for women where she would likely see muscle definition. 14-20% is the athletic range where muscle definition would be really obvious.

Now, most at-home scales that also measure body fat are not overly reliable. Most of these scales use something called biometric impedance.

> The bioimpedance scale uses a very low voltage electrical circuit (we promise it doesn't hurt!) that goes from your toes all the way to your head. Muscle and fat conduct electricity at different rates, so the bioimpedance scale can show us the difference between how much muscle and fat our patients have[17]. - Johns Hopkins Medicine on Bioimpedance scales

Here's a really important distinction I had to get comfortable with towards the beginning: knowing that these scales are not incredibly reliable or accurate, the number they produce isn't necessarily your actual body fat percentage. It's less important — for me — to know the actual number and more important for me to follow the trends. Let's say that my scale told me I was

---

[17] Johns Hopkins Medicine on Bioimpedance scales:
https://www.hopkinsmedicine.org/all-childrens-hospital/services/pediatric-and-adolescent-medicine/healthy-weight-initiative/resources-for-all-ages/bioimpedance-scale-in-children

20% body fat and then a month later it told me that I was 18% body fat. Whether I'm actually 20% and then 18% is less relevant than what is more likely true: I was losing fat; regardless of the number.

There are a variety of different types of ways to measure body fat. Home scales are often the most affordable if you want a scale. There's also something called skinfold calibers. One of these looks like a giant clamp thing. You use it to pinch your skin in a few different places. When you pinch your skin it essentially measures in millimeters how thick your skin is in those various places. There are standard places people measure (chest for men, abdomen, thigh, etc). They usually come with a table that allows you to look up, based on your age and weight, what your body fat percentage is. This method also has a few limitations: it is hard to do on yourself (but not impossible) and you need to measure in consistent places. The results could vary based on your hydration levels (measuring first thing in the morning vs after you've been drinking liquids for a while will affect the results). It also has no way to measure visceral fat. A pair of skinfold calipers is pretty inexpensive.

There are much more expensive options like something called a DEXA scan. This is essentially an X-ray machine that can detect body fat percentage, bone density, and a bunch of other metrics. You probably don't have this in your home and they can cost around $150 per scan. While they can be very accurate, it's not likely this is a thing you're going to do very often.

For someone who loves data as much as I do, all of this was both fascinating and overwhelming to learn about. Aside from the periodic bloodwork I was getting done to check my cholesterol, my body fat percentage trends became the best metric for me to track because a body fat percentage that was trending down could be correlated with lowered inflammation in my body which helps to reduce cholesterol, better insulin sensitivity which helps to reduce triglycerides. A lower body fat percentage also usually means more muscle mass. More muscle mass means my body will have better glucose regulation which also helps to manage triglycerides. There isn't a direct correlation between lower body fat percentages and improved cholesterol but there's definitely an indirect connection.

In case you were wondering — yes — I use the scale *and* the skinfold calipers. For me, the skinfold calipers also present a lower body fat percentage than the scale. I take the value of both and average them out to give me, perhaps unreasonably, a slightly more accurate number. Still, the number for me is less important than the trends.

4

Do you know what else is helpful regarding progress? Photos. Take a photo of yourself, but not every day, in the same position and at roughly the same time. Given that we've already established that progress doesn't happen overnight and the expectations that we set or that are set for us are generally not always close to the actual realistic progress, having photos that are spaced out over time is a great way for you to actually see if your body has changed. If you're the person who does 15 bicep curls and then looks in the mirror to see if your arm muscle got bigger (and you know you've done it), I have news for you: it didn't. However, if you've been working out a lot and you look at a picture of yourself from a month ago vs today, you might actually see a difference. I will talk more about this in Part Four but trust me: seeing the progress isn't about vanity. It is reassuring and makes you feel good and is therefore worth doing.

While these physical metrics provided tangible evidence of change, they told only part of the story. Just as body composition offers a deeper truth than weight alone, psychological progress reveals itself in ways that aren't always easily measured.

So let's talk about psychological progress.

What is the equivalent of healthy cholesterol or better muscle tone or losing 10 pounds as it relates to your mental health? I've sat staring at the computer screen for quite a while trying to figure out how to articulate how I've measured my own progress on this front. It's very challenging. There was no single moment — like if I ran a mile in under 10 minutes — where I could say, "This is progress."

I do, however, remember a handful of moments in the course of this journey that I think fall under the umbrella of mental health progress; or are at least related. Let's start with the photo I shared in Chapter 5 with my friend:

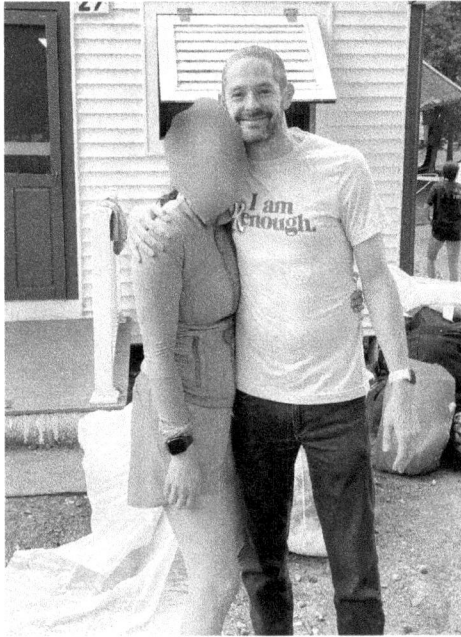

When my friend sent me this photo, while I could objectively see abdominal muscles in the photo, my first reaction was actually to feel self-conscious. I was uncomfortable. Was my shirt too tight? Were other people noticing? Do people think I'm showing off?

Even though it's reasonable to have known what I looked like before and then to see this photo and think it was a net positive change, it still made me feel weird at the time. It made me feel a sense of shame.

5

Somewhere along the way, however, it stopped feeling weird. I stopped worrying about what other people might think and started focusing on what made me feel comfortable. This, I think, is related to the types — or rather the sizes — of clothes I was wearing. You know the game where you talk to your friends about what superpower you'd have if you could choose any? Some people choose the ability to fly while others choose invisibility. My superpower has always been to fit into whatever clothes are on the mannequin at the clothes store. This has always been an incredibly helpful "skill" because I don't have a good sense of style (I also "suffer" as someone who is color-deficient[18]).

I know that whoever styled the mannequins has a better sense of style than I do. Because I basically have the same dimensions as the mannequin (although I have a head), I can just take whatever it's wearing and even if I can't describe what colors it is, I have a reasonable chance of it looking good.

The shift in my clothing choices marked more than just a change in size — it reflected a fundamental change in how I saw myself. Where I once used loose shirts as camouflage, I began choosing clothes that actually fit. This wasn't about showing off — it was about stopping the habit of hiding. The mannequin that had once been my style guide became a symbol of how I'd used *fine* as an excuse to avoid attention. Now, even with my color deficiency making style choices challenging, I found myself making intentional choices about how I presented myself rather than defaulting to whatever would help me blend in.

---

[18] Color deficiency is not color blindness. I can see color. I just can't always define which color I'm seeing. Someone with red-green color blindness, for example, can't see that those are different colors. I can see that they are two different colors, but I can't always tell you which is red and which is green.

So I don't worry about style all that much. I worry about being comfortable. Here's the thing: during the dadbod phase of my life, I was wearing a lot of medium and some large-sized shirts. My pants — jeans mostly — were always the same size. The clothes seemed to fit me ... fine. Once I started getting healthier and my body started to change, I started feeling like I looked like my clothes were way too big. The shirts that I had made me look like someone put a shrinking spell on me. I was essentially swimming in the large shirts and even in some of the mediums. I slowly started replacing my clothes with smaller sizes. This naturally made things fit a little tighter but were much more comfortable for me because I didn't feel like someone put me in a clothes dryer and I shrunk (even if I had). It never crossed my mind that anyone would notice.

6

There was another time, more recently, I was at a meeting in my town and someone came up to me who had only known me for a handful of recent years and therefore only known me in dadbod form. After the meeting, she approached me and asked if I was ok. Was I eating enough? A different reaction triggered in me this time. This time, instead of feeling uncomfortable or self-conscious like I had before, I got defensive in my own head. How could this person not recognize that what she had seen before was the "not ok" version of me and now what she was seeing was the result of a lot of hard work and discipline? With the first example I used, I felt some shame and now I believe the defensive reaction I had was because I actually was feeling pride. I wasn't ashamed anymore. I wasn't uncomfortable. That is progress.

Social situations became another measure of progress. At the hot Pilates studio, I evolved from the guy who kept his shirt on despite the heat to someone who could focus on the workout rather than others' perceptions. In conversations about health and fitness, I shifted from deflecting to engaging. When friends or colleagues commented on changes, I learned to accept their observations without immediately explaining them away. These weren't conscious decisions — they were evidence of progress I only recognized in retrospect.

The real measurement of psychological progress isn't in dramatic moments but in these subtle shifts — from hiding to existing comfortably, from shame to acceptance, from deflection to engagement. While you can't plot these changes on a graph, they're just as real as any drop in triglycerides.

These two moments — the t-shirt photo and the concerned question — show how psychological progress isn't linear but cyclical. Each new situation tests our growth. The first time someone noticed my changes, I wanted to hide. The second time, I felt defensive pride. That shift from shame to pride wasn't just emotional — it manifested in concrete ways. I started selecting clothes that fit properly instead of hiding in oversized shirts. I spoke more openly about my fitness journey instead of deflecting comments. When people asked about my changes, I began sharing the work behind them rather than minimizing the achievement.

The real metric of psychological progress isn't feeling perfectly confident — it's how quickly we recover from moments of self-doubt. While physical progress shows up in blood tests and body fat measurements, mental progress appears in these subtle shifts of reaction and behavior. There's no scale for measuring increased comfort in your own skin, but you know it when you feel it.

***

Something to think about...

What's one thing you feel self-conscious

about?

CHAPTER NINE

THE TORTOISE CHOICE

1

Everyone knows the story of the tortoise and the hare. The tortoise wins through steady progress while the hare, overconfident in his natural speed, loses by trying to take shortcuts. It's a simple lesson we've all heard since childhood. Yet somehow, when it comes to health and fitness, we keep trying to be the hare.

I used to think I was immune to marketing hype. As someone who writes code as a software engineer for a living, I pride myself on logic and critical thinking. Yet there I was, scrolling through social media, pausing on posts about "revolutionary" workout programs and "game-changing" supplements. Maybe this pre-workout powder would be the edge I needed. Maybe this 30-day challenge would fast-track my progress. The fitness industry isn't just selling products — it's selling the dream of being the hare in a tortoise's journey.

Of course, everyone would prefer to move as quickly as the hare; it just isn't usually possible if you want to actually achieve your goals. I covered unrealistic expectation setting in chapter 7. In this chapter, we'll explore the influence of social media — and marketing in general — on health and fitness culture.

The fitness and health industry has mastered the art of selling transformation. Every January, gym memberships have an enrollment spike. Magazine covers promise "New Year, New You." Social media feeds fill up with before-and-after photos and discount codes for miracle supplements. It's a $100 billion industry that caters to many of our biggest insecurities.

But why does it work so well? Perhaps because, unlike many other skills or achievements, fitness and health feel accessible. We all have bodies. We've probably all exercised at some point in our lives. How hard could it be to transform ourselves if we just find the right program, the right supplement, or the right influencer to follow? If you call now, we'll send you a second Thigh Master for FREE (plus shipping and handling)!

2

The marketing for this industry also does a great job of leaning into the "need" vs "want" positioning. You might want that air fryer that has WiFi connectivity and can detect what food is inside and automatically determine how long to cook it for but even you know — when you see the commercial on TV — that you don't need it. Good health though? We all know we need that. The easier that is to achieve the more likely I'll be to jump on board. There's a bonus in the marketing too: you can start right now. It's easy.

This combination of urgent need and promised quick results creates a unique blind spot in our critical thinking. The same person who would laugh at the idea of performing surgery after watching Grey's Anatomy would probably confidently attempt a complete fitness transformation after watching a few TikTok videos.

Unlike flying a fighter jet or performing surgery, the barrier to entry feels nonexistent. You don't need special equipment, years of training, or someone's permission to try that 8-minute abs video. You just need a floor. The combination of what seems very accessible and apparent simplicity creates a dangerous illusion — if the actions look easy to replicate, surely the results must be too. I don't blame them. They are selling a product in the same way that all products get sold. In the same way that you might shop around and do research when it's time to buy a new car or a new TV — looking for what will provide you with the result you are interested in — you should probably do that same research before you get sucked into a fitness sales pitch. I see them too and am definitely susceptible to their charms. But why?

3

It brings me back to when I was a kid watching Saturday morning GI Joe and Transformers cartoons. It was inevitable that during the commercials I'd see something about a new toy that looked like so much fun. At that age, I had no way to self-regulate or temper the excitement. I needed that new He-Man toy right this second. Or when my grandmother would give me the Toys R' Us circular before Hanukkah each year so I could circle the toys I wanted and everything looked like so much fun so I circled everything. Just like when I was a kid, when it came to toys my eyes were always bigger than my stomach. Getting ALL the toys was not realistic but that's what I wanted! It was effective marketing then and it's effective marketing now. That industry knows exactly what we want to see and they also know WHO should show it to us:

Someone who is in great shape. Be honest for a second: if you saw a doctor who was really overweight, would you question their credibility? How could they possibly be able to help me be healthy if they aren't healthy themselves? They might be the nicest person in the world and more importantly in this context, the most competent doctor. I'm not suggesting they aren't either of those things. I'm suggesting that I (and perhaps you) would have a bit of an inner dialog questioning that competency just by looking at them. I know that's not fair — but I suspect that it's probably true.

4

Do you know all the people you see in fitness advertising? They are all in incredible shape. They're shredded. You see those people and think that it doesn't even matter what they're selling; you're in because if you just do whatever it is that they're telling you, you can *look* just like them. For many people, the product they are selling isn't the Thigh Master, the Ab Roller, the Soloflex, or this diet or that diet or this supplement or that supplement. They are selling a version of themselves. Listen to what they're saying and you can be just like them. But again, why? What is about *them* that's so desirable? Why do I feel the need to be like them?

Have you ever seen the movie Top Gun? When you left the theater did you feel confident that you could land an F-14 fighter jet on the deck of the USS Enterprise? Are you qualified to be a trial lawyer because you just binged the first 32 seasons of Law & Order? I played the video game Guitar Hero a bunch of years ago and now — because of that — I'm headlining at Coachella. There was also this time that I delivered a baby in an elevator after telling the woman who was in labor that it was ok, I had watched every episode of ER. Why is it that the cheeseburger I just made looks awful — even after I took notes while watching Bobby Flay make the best-looking cheeseburger I've ever seen while competing on Iron Chef? I just wish Simon Cowell could hear me sing while I was in the shower or driving alone. I'd definitely be the next American Idol.

These are all ridiculous examples. Here's one more ridiculous example: I see a 30-second fitness reel and think: "Yeah, I could look like that in a few weeks." Why do we apply logical thinking to these other skills but suspend it for fitness? We've all been there: it's 1:00 am, you can't sleep, and somehow you're watching a guy with impossibly defined muscle tone tell you that you're just six minutes away, 3 days a week, from looking like him. The infomercial promises it's "just that easy." The before-and-after photos are compelling. The testimonials are convincing. And great news, it's only four easy payments of $29.99. Wait! If you call they'll knock one of those payments off!

We've all done it: scrolled through fitness influencer posts thinking 'Why don't I look like that?' while conveniently forgetting that:

- This is literally their full-time job

- They're probably quite a bit younger than I am

- The perfect after photo probably took 47 takes

- They have professional photographers, lighting, and an Adobe Photoshop license.

Here I was, a software engineer and dad in his forties, comparing myself to a 28-year-old professional fitness influencer whose job is working out and being the subject of professional photographers. It's like wondering why my Chef Boyardee canned ravioli doesn't look like a professional chef's — we're not playing the same game. Just like I wouldn't want George Clooney performing actual surgery (although I could be convinced) after playing a doctor on TV, maybe I shouldn't expect to look like @FitnessGuru247 after watching their TikTok tutorials.

But why do we keep falling for it? The answer lies deeper than just clever marketing or social media filters. There's something about fitness transformation that taps into our hopes, insecurities, and desire for quick change in a way other skills don't.

5

When we see a fitness transformation, we're not just seeing physical change — we're told that what we're seeing is a promise of becoming a "better" version of ourselves. That pull is stronger than any late-night infomercial or doom-scrolling on TikTok could achieve alone. Unlike learning to fly or practicing law, fitness transformation feels like unlocking something already within us. It's not about learning new skills — it's about revealing our "true" potential. It feels very reaffirming.

The fitness and health industry has mastered linking physical transformation to personal identity. "The best version of you" isn't just about muscle tone — it's about confidence, success, and self-actualization. When an influencer shows their transformation, they're not just displaying physical changes. They're showing career success, maybe even relationship happiness, and life fulfillment — all seemingly unlocked through fitness and just taking a few easy steps.

This narrative is powerful because it suggests that our "best self" is already within us, just waiting to be revealed through the right program, supplement, or workout routine. It's almost like I don't need to learn anything new — I just need to refine what I already do. It's uncovering what's already there. And who wouldn't want that version of themselves?

I think there's also often a moment of realization. I do believe we tell ourselves that while "I'll never actually look like that person," maybe [looks over shoulder to see if anyone is looking] if I do just like, some of that, I could get pretty close to whatever that person is putting on display. I've told myself that of course, I don't want to be a fitness influencer. That's not me. I'm a software engineer. Given that, I don't need to work as hard as that person probably worked for as long as that person worked.

THE PARADOX OF FINE

I can do much less and get sufficient results much faster. The focus starts to shift from *what I want to do* to *how fast can I do it.*

This act of rationalization leads you even deeper into the marketing hole and further into the mindset of the hare.

6

In Chapter 7 I used the 5k example to demonstrate an unfortunately all-too-common example of pushing ourselves too quickly and the physical risks associated with that. Sometimes when my wife and I go out for dinner, she'll order a dirty martini. This is a beverage presentation I will never understand. With the acknowledgment that I'm not a drinker of alcohol and do not understand much about that genre of beverage, I can not wrap my head around why martini glasses *must* be filled all the way to the rim of the glass. Logically, just maybe put slightly less liquid in or if the amount of liquid is so important, make the glass a little bit taller. Watching someone serve a martini in a restaurant is one of the more absurd circus acts you can witness. There's always liquid spilling over the edge or on the tray or on the floor or down your hands. By the time the glass gets to the table — even if you have the best server — the glass is now a bit emptier — which it probably should have been, to begin with. Of course, some servers have a cheat code. They bring the empty glass to the table and one of those shaker things. They pour the martini into the glass at the table so they don't have to risk moving it. The responsibility shifts to the consumer.

If you try to move that glass too quickly the liquid will spill. In addition, there's too much liquid in it, so the risk of a spill is even greater.

Your fitness and health goals work the same way. Less liquid in the martini glass is like having smaller and more achievable goals. Not rushing to try and achieve those goals is like taking the extra time to walk with the filled martini glass as if you're balancing an egg on your head in your high school physics class. There are very few things that I do in life that are — or work — better *because* I rushed through them.

The physical risks of rushing are a bit more apparent. If I was to try and do a back squat with a barbell and load more weight than I probably should because I feel confident in my ability even if I've not practiced the proper form or built up to that weight, I'm much more likely to hurt myself. It's so easy to forget about your weightlifting form because that part is much less "fun" and the stories we hear related to building muscle involve "lifting heavy" and don't often talk about proper form so I focus on lifting heavy and not on doing it properly.

Once I hurt myself — and I will — there are downstream impacts: I have to stop lifting entirely. This throws off my energy for the day because I've gotten accustomed to working out in some form each day. In whatever recovery time I need to heal, I start feeling anxious about losing progress because this whole thing was predicated on "going fast." It's really hard to sit still and go fast at the same time. Now I start to feel like I'm failing. The physical problem turns into a psychological one. Once I start to feel a little better — but not fully healed — I tell myself I better get started again because I'm anxious to minimize the progress loss. It's now pretty common for people to go right back to where they were before they got hurt because they either write off the injury-causing moment as a fluke or feel like they have to make up for lost time. The risk of injury is even higher now because I am not fully healed, I'm still driven by speed and I have the added stress of feeling like I'm falling behind.

What's actually happening now is that my desire to go quickly makes it much more likely that it will actually take longer to attain my goals — if I can at all — than if I had just gone slower and been more deliberate from the beginning.

Rushing potentially leads to injury. Injury likely leads to anxiety — or at the very least disappointment. That anxiety and/or disappointment often leads to rushing back. This is a pretty harmful loop.

7

This cycle doesn't just take a physical toll — it damages our relationship with fitness itself. Each rushed attempt followed by a setback makes us more desperate for quick fixes, have less confidence in the plan, and therefore more susceptible to marketing promises or anything that we think will give us a leg up. We start viewing fitness as a sprint rather than a journey, making each "failure" compound and feel more devastating. This starts to feel like "I keep trying and nothing is working."

But there's freedom in choosing to be the tortoise. When you remove the pressure of speed, you create space to actually enjoy the process which in and of itself makes it more likely that you'll be successful. Small, consistent progress might not make for dramatic social media posts, but it builds something more valuable: sustainable change that becomes part of who you are rather than something you're rushing to achieve.

I also don't think that all or even most influencers — and marketing in general — in the health and fitness space are bad. I believe they believe that what they're telling us is effective and it very well may be for some people. It may even ultimately be effective for you. It's probably safe to assume that the person doing the selling isn't at the same level of progress or the same place on their own journey's timeline as you are. They have likely had years of working on themselves to get to where they feel like they can actually sell something. If you were getting on a flight somewhere and were given the choice of two pilots would you choose the pilot who just got their pilot's license but assures you that they've spent years playing Microsoft's Flight Simulator game or the pilot who has actually flown real passenger planes for 15 years? I'm guessing you'd choose the more experienced pilot. So would I. Now, if you walked up to the plane and saw that one of the engines was dangling off the wing and the other engine was on fire, you'd probably decide that this flight was not right for you regardless of who was flying.

There's nothing wrong with buying that ab roller or trying that supplement so long as you do the proper research and maybe even speak to a professional who is familiar with your circumstances. The person on the other side of your phone screen doesn't know you. They don't understand your life or your complexities and certainly not your medical history. Maybe those things will end up being right for you but please don't take their word for it at face value just because they say so. We're all different people with different needs.

The fitness industry will always try to sell speed — fitness's version of Oreos — and our natural inclination will always be to buy it. But real transformation — the kind that lasts — happens at the speed of *your* adaptation and not marketing. The tortoise wins not just because slow and steady progress works, but because it builds something marketing can't sell: sustainable change that becomes part of who you are.

Remember: that filled martini glass gets to your table a lot faster and fuller when the server doesn't rush trying to get it there.

The evidence of this approach for me wasn't the before-and-after photos; it's in the lasting changes that transformed more than my body, but also the way I felt about myself.

***

Something to think about...

What quick fixes have you tried and how did they go?

PART FOUR

UNEXPECTED DISCOVERIES

CHAPTER TEN

SPEAKING UP

1

Transformation doesn't happen in isolation. As my relationship with health evolved and my body changed, I noticed other changes beginning to surface. The confidence that came from achieving things I hadn't considered or for those things I did consider, what once seemed way out of reach started spilling into other areas of my life. I found myself wanting to share my story and experiences, not just about fitness, but about all the unexpected discoveries along the way.

When I first started this journey, the last thing I expected was that I'd end up writing about it. As someone who seems to have been dealing with hidden body image issues for decades, the idea of openly discussing health and fitness would have seemed absurd. Yet here I was, finding myself in conversations about cholesterol numbers, nutrition, and workout routines, sharing what I'd learned about the gap between expectations and reality.

It wasn't about becoming some fitness guru or health expert — I'm far from either. It was about recognizing that my struggles and discoveries might resonate with others who were also trying to navigate their own journey past "fine" even if they didn't know it either. I found a community.

What started as solitary early morning workouts and trying to simply eat better gradually evolved into conversations with others on similar journeys. Each shared struggle or small victory created connections I never sought out before. I initially just wanted to lower my cholesterol but now found myself part of something bigger and more interesting. In the previous chapter I explored the influence of marketing and things we see on social media. At the beginning of my journey, the risk of those things influencing my process was much higher and outsized for me because I hadn't yet discovered the community of people in my life who were also interested in the same things as me. We might have had different goals, different life situations, and different circumstances in general but what we had in common — if you abstract out the specifics — was that we're all trying to get healthier.

It is so much more interesting and fun to be part of a larger community. Some of what allowed it to be fun is that my confidence grew. As I learned more about how to do the things that would benefit me and my goals along with the things that I enjoyed doing, Now the influencers, the podcasts, and the blog posts were just more research. In the beginning — because I didn't have the confidence or knowledge to figure out what I needed for myself — I took what I heard from the people with millions of listeners or followers as dogma.

I knew that I was supposed to do things like deadlifts, bench presses, and squats. Those are great compound lifts; possibly the three best. I knew I was supposed to eat broccoli and asparagus. Looking back, it felt similar to the research and stories I heard when my wife was pregnant with our first daughter. The problem back then was similar to the problem now: we're all different and there is rarely a one-size-fits-all prescription for how fitness, health, or even parenting should work. The advice really is just a set of loose guidelines that can help inform you. Ultimately it is up to you to figure out what works for you and the best way to do that is to learn from as many different sources as possible and to gain experience.

As Fred Rogers said in the context of seeing scary things: "Look for the helpers. You will always find people who are helping." I apply that in a more general sense than I believe Mr. Rogers intended but I think it still works. I haven't been successful as a parent without my wife. I haven't been successful in my career without my co-workers. I wasn't going to be successful in this without my doctor, my trainer, my family supporting me, my friends going through similar experiences, *and* the vast resources available broadly. I wasn't going to be successful without a community.

2

The confidence to be comfortable knowing you don't really know what you're doing and then being willing to seek out help was the beginning of something else for me. As I started to really get interested in learning more about what it would take to make me healthier it sparked a new urge to be creative in other ways.

I've always been the type of person who enjoys learning new things. I have always enjoyed watching the Discovery Channel or how things get made. Other than my career as a software engineer, I never really had the urge to make anything. But then I did. When my daughters were born I started writing a blog about my parenting experience. I always enjoyed writing and the various things my daughters were experiencing seemed like a good excuse to stretch that writing muscle. I wrote about potty training, sleep schedules, and learning how to read. I wrote about going to kindergarten, experiencing death, and even the infamous sex talk. As my daughters got older — into their teenage years — my writing frequency started to diminish. I started feeling like the things I wanted to write about that were age-appropriate for my daughters were not my business to share.

I decided I had to stop writing that blog but still wanted to write. For around a decade I had been tinkering with the idea of writing a book because I thought it would be fun and another interesting thing to learn how to do. I could never figure out how to get it off the ground. I kept starting and stopping. Nothing felt right. Deciding to end the blog was probably something I was ok with because I was feeling particularly creative. I was hungry to try my hand at something new. When I was working through the mental gymnastics about how to end the blog, it all clicked. Write a book about my parenting experience. That book, "Nature & Nurture: A Journey Through the Fog of Parenting," was published in August of 2024.

My desire to express myself creatively sparked and grew at the same time that I was starting to feel confident about my improved health and fitness. I can't imagine that was a coincidence. As I was writing "Nature & Nurture," I had no idea what I was doing. It was an exciting process that involved a lot of conversations with a lot of people who knew more about how to write and publish a book than I did (sounds familiar). I learned a ton. I had always figured that once that book was written and then published, the creative itch would be scratched. It wasn't.

I'd say around 75% of the way through writing "Nature & Nurture" I started feeling like I had three other ideas to write about. I figured I'd give myself some time off and then when I figured out which of the ideas made the most sense to me I'd start to work on an outline. This book was one of those ideas and I'm typing *this* word less than four months after my first book was published. The desire to express myself has grown like a cartoon snowball rolling down a hill. If not for the confidence I've felt since making — and seeing — progress with my health and fitness journey, I don't think the first book would have happened and this book certainly wouldn't have.

3

The lessons from this journey started appearing in unexpected places. The same patience I learned to apply to fitness progress helped me tackle long-term projects at work. Understanding that transformation takes time made me a more methodical problem-solver. Even my approach to learning new technologies shifted — I stopped expecting instant mastery and started appreciating the process.

The gym taught me that showing up consistently matters more than occasional heroic efforts. This translated directly to writing — daily progress, even small amounts, accomplished more than sporadic marathon sessions. The discipline of tracking progress, whether in workout logs or blood work results, showed up in how I approached other goals.

Perhaps most importantly, I learned that growth in any area rarely happens in isolation. Just as physical training also improved my mental strength, each new challenge I tackled made the next one feel more achievable. Success bred success, creating a momentum that carried beyond just health and fitness.

Each small win — whether in the gym, writing, or life — builds belief in what's possible. The patterns became more clear as I learned and experienced more: set realistic goals, track progress, and adjust the plan based on results. Like compound exercises that work multiple muscle groups, each new challenge strengthened multiple aspects of life. Writing built discipline. Discipline built consistency. Consistency built results. Results motivated repetition of the process.

What started as a mission to lower cholesterol had expanded into something much broader. The tools and mindset that worked for health goals proved equally valuable elsewhere. Progress in one area created confidence to pursue growth in others. The most powerful realization wasn't about physical transformation at all — it was understanding that growth compounds. Just as regular exercise builds strength over time, regular challenges build capability. Each new challenge felt less daunting because I'd proven to myself that sustainable change was possible.

Writing a book seemed impossible until it wasn't. Publishing seemed out of reach until it happened. Each achievement wasn't just a singular success — it was evidence that other *impossible* goals might be achievable too. The boundaries of what felt possible kept expanding, not because the challenges got easier, but because I got better at facing them.

When you start on your journey, regardless of what goals you set for yourself — large or small — there will inevitably be things that you can't predict because you just don't have the frame of reference. When my daughters were infants, if I asked them who was going to win the World Series that year they'd just stare at me and then probably drool all over a thick cardboard board book. How would they have any idea about the World Series at that age? They had no frame of reference.

I have this long-standing story I like to tell myself about skydiving. You can be the most prepared person in the world. You can sit on the tarmac with your parachute and you can pack it and unpack it a bunch of times. You can check every strap and every lock and every pocket. Here's the thing though: you won't truly know if the parachute will really work until you jump out of the plane from up in the sky. All the preparation in the world won't provide you with more information than actually experiencing it. Of course, I hope for your sake that the parachute opens.

I often apply the concept to hiring other engineers at work. I can interview people with the best of them. I have great questions that I'm quite proud of. The team will vet a candidate for technical competency and see if they'd be a good fit for the company culture. We can make sure that the candidate's compensation ask is in line with what the company pays. We can do background checks and reference checks and all the diligence that's available. None of that guarantees that the person will actually be a great member of the team. You won't know that until they get there and start working.

This type of journey — the one to get healthier — works the same way. You can (and should) have a goal in mind. You can (and should) research and plan and figure out how you're going to approach achieving the goal. Just like skydiving — hopefully without the risk of catastrophic disaster — and just like hiring a new employee, you'll learn more from actually experiencing it than you will from thinking about experiencing it. Nobody can tell you exactly how to do this. Nobody should pack this particular parachute for you. While you can (and should) seek out help and learn as much as you can from as many people as possible, ultimately you're the one who has to jump out of that plane.

Who knows what you'll discover about yourself along the way so pull the ripcord.

There's a movie called "Contact" that came out in 1997. It stars Jodie Foster as a character named Ellie Arroway. I can't remember much about the movie but there was one scene near the end that struck me as particularly interesting. Ellie is in a space-travel ship of sorts to seek out extraterrestrial life based on a radio signal she found. In the scene, she's harnessed into a flight chair for safety. As the scene progresses, she (and the camera) are experiencing a heavy amount of turbulence from the journey through some sort of sequence of wormholes. At one point she sees a small compass on a necklace gently floating in front of her. She has a realization (one that the audience doesn't quite get yet). She disengages the harness for her chair and immediately starts to gently float in the middle of the ship while the chair continues its turbulent rattle. She is now completely still.

It might be a stretch but this feels applicable to my journey. Sitting in that chair, safely harnessed in, felt like the logical thing to do. Everything we know is that you should be buckled in for safety. It was not until Dr. Ellie Arroway learned something about her environment — something she didn't previously know or consider — that she was truly free to achieve her goal. She literally released herself from the seat and metaphorically released herself from being held back. She just didn't know it until she was experiencing it.

Like Dr. Arroway, we often stay strapped into what feels safe and logical, not realizing that releasing ourselves from those constraints might be exactly what we need. My journey started with cholesterol numbers but led to discoveries I couldn't have predicted or prepared for. Yours will likely be different but that's the point — you won't know what's possible until you unstrap yourself from *fine* and start floating freely in your own direction.

***

Something to think about...

How comfortable are you sharing your

goals with others? What support system

could help you succeed?

CHAPTER ELEVEN

THE MIRROR MOMENT

1

There's a moment that most people on a fitness journey know: standing in front of the bathroom mirror, noticing changes in your body, and then maybe feeling the slightest bit conflicted about those changes. I think I'm proud of what I've accomplished so far. Is feeling proud just a form of vanity in this regard? Is that pride making me feel self-conscious? Is it a shame that makes us minimize our progress? The mirror reflects more than just physical transformation — it reflects our complicated relationship with self-improvement.

My initial goal had nothing to do with my body or physical appearance. I had no goal for how much weight I wanted to be able to lift. Despite those things, here I was, noticing changes in my body that I hadn't expected and feeling a sense of pride that I had never felt before followed by metaphorically looking around to make sure nobody else could see that I had noticed myself. It could have been simple. I could have just participated in a bit of self-talk and said, "Matt, nice job — keep working." Nope. Not me. I found myself in an internal debate that ultimately boiled down to this: is it ok for me to be proud of what I've accomplished so far and if so, what is the appropriate way to express it?

My first instinct was to think, "Yes," it's not only ok for me to be proud of what I'd accomplished so far but I'd argue that it was appropriate. We should celebrate our victories; however large or small. The second part is where I find I often get hung up. What is the appropriate way to express it? There are a variety of ways — some healthy and some less so — one might express pride in themselves or something they've done but *pride* isn't just a five-letter word.

When I figure out a smart way to solve some tough software engineering problem, I feel proud. When I got elected to my town's school board, I felt proud. When I saw the first blood test results in September of 2021 and my triglycerides had come down, I felt proud. I think it's ok to objectively look at an accomplishment and feel good about it. I feel proud because *I* worked hard and accomplished something. Is there a way to share that pride? When does pride become vanity?

I think there's a subtle distinction. The line is very blurry and completely subjective. If I solve a tough software engineering problem and then make an effort to make sure that everyone on my team knows that *I* did it, that feels like vanity. In that case, it's not about the solution to the problem, it's purely about having people recognize that I was the one who solved it.

If you've ever been to one of the big-box chain gyms, you've probably seen the person (almost always a guy) who finishes a workout or even just one particular exercise and then goes and poses in front of the mirror. Let's assume for the sake of this exercise that the person is not about to compete in a bodybuilding or fitness competition and needs to practice their posing. It's probably safe to assume that in that context, doing some flexing in the wall-to-wall mirror of a giant room filled with other people might be skewed a bit towards attention-seeking. At that point, it's not that the person worked hard to get the physique that they have but rather that they want *you* to see it. That feels like vanity to me.

A challenge here is that people — and I include myself in that group — do want to share their success with others. It's a good feeling to have someone else recognize your hard work. We don't typically live on islands stranded all alone. We're social creatures who often seek validation from the people around us. I think there's also a bit of a sanity check. Is what I'm seeing in the mirror real or just in my head? Maybe if someone I trust recognizes it too, that will validate that what I'm seeing isn't skewed by my own perception. There is a paradox or at the very least some grey area. How do I reconcile the desire that we all share to want to get validation from people beyond who we see in the mirror but do so in a way that I — and they — don't feel like I'm bragging or being vain?

There's also an interesting set of double standards for men and women in the fitness area (and in plenty of other areas). Let's explore those in general terms:

Again, these are generalizations.

A "manly" man is supposed to be strong but not care too much about their appearance. Women should want to look fit but definitely not show it. Too much muscle on a woman is not "feminine" enough. Women who show pride in their fitness are criticized. Men who show pride in their fitness are praised. As a result, women are more likely to minimize their fitness achievements to appear modest.

So how much pride is acceptable? How much vanity?

2

These gender differences aren't just anecdotal. Research shows significant disparities in how men and women process and display fitness achievements. Women face conflicting messages: be fit but not too fit, be proud but not show it, care about appearance but don't appear to care too much. Men face different but equally complicated expectations: be strong but don't be vain about it, care about fitness but maintain an air of effortlessness.

Here's another general statistic about gender differences as they relate to body image and body satisfaction : women who experience body dissatisfaction (and it's a lot of women) have a primary desire to lose some weight. Men who experience body dissatisfaction (not quite as high as women) have a primary desire to be more muscular[19]. As a man, I'm supposed to be able to lift

---

[19] From the National Eating Disorders Association:
https://www.nationaleatingdisorders.org/body-image-and-eating-disorders/

more weight, be stronger, and not be too thin (or heaven forbid, skinny). As a woman, you're supposed to be thin, not be too strong (or heaven forbid, too muscular).

Now I'm getting somewhere. My whole life, I was "the skinny kid." I never matched up with the generalized stereotype of what a "man" was supposed to look like.

Do you know the word ectomorph? There are 3 different body types: ectomorphs, mesomorphs, and endomorphs. Let's talk about the differences because I think it will create some useful context.

- Ectomorphs are characterized by a slim body frame, small shoulders and hips, long arms and legs, and less muscle mass. They have relatively smaller muscles relative to bone length. Often have a fast metabolism which makes it difficult to gain mass.

- Mesomorphs are characterized by a medium build with higher-than-average muscular development, a low body fat percentage, broad shoulders, and a muscular chest, shoulders, and limbs. They typically have a very efficient metabolism and can gain or lose mass more easily.

- Endomorphs are characterized by a larger, rounder body shape, high levels of body fat, a propensity to gain weight, and shorter arms and legs. They have a slower metabolism.

I was never aware of these different body type categorizations but once I knew these definitions existed, it really helped me to understand my body. I am definitely an ectomorph.

Constitution of the human body

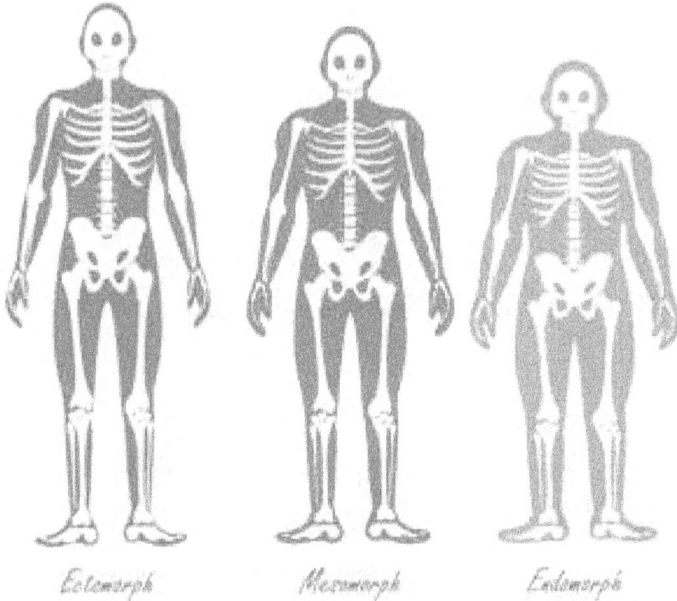

Ectomorph   Mesomorph   Endomorph

Credit: National Academy of Sports Medicine[20]

Men who identify as "naturally thin" often experience unique psychological challenges. While society celebrates thinness in women, men who are "skinny" often face different social pressures and expectations. Being "the skinny kid" wasn't just about social perception — it was about my fundamental body type. Ectomorphs, characterized by naturally lean builds and faster metabolisms, often struggle to gain muscle mass. Understanding this wasn't just about putting a label on being

---

[20] NASM body types: https://www.nasm.org/resource-center/blog/body-types-how-to-train-diet-for-your-body-type?srsltid=AfmBOopbpJzVNjCrF7NLWPnd1U0LJcZQBd5XWt2rqhrPZj3e9YA-LPVk

skinny — it helped explain why my body responded differently to exercise and nutrition than others'.

It turns out that there are different ways you might train depending on your body type and your goals. According to the National Academy of Sports Medicine[21], Endomorphs "maximize calorie burn and the improvement of metabolic efficiency by primarily using high-intensity, metabolic training techniques" and "consume a high-protein diet with balanced carbs and fats that maintains a slight negative energy balance."

Mesomorphs "Eat specifically for fitness goals and activity, increasing or decreasing daily calories to preferentially control body composition with positive, neutral, or negative energy balances" and "Increase protein intakes to as high as 2.2 grams per kilogram of body weight for muscle gain goals; or, keep closer to the 0.8 gram per kilogram of body weight FDA recommended dietary allowance (RDA) when healthy body composition maintenance is all that is desired."

Ectomorphs (like me) "Maximize muscle gain using lower-intensity hypertrophy and maximal strength resistance training with longer rest periods" and "Consume a high-protein diet with balanced carbs and fats that maintains a positive energy balance." Hypertrophy, by the way, means increasing muscle size through targeted training as you increase volume over time. You are essentially damaging your muscles so that your body can repair them and they come back bigger. This is not the same thing as

---

[21] NASM How to train as an endomorph: https://www.nasm.org/resource-center/blog/body-types-how-to-train-diet-for-your-body-type?srsltid=AfmBOopbpJzVNjCrF7NLWPnd1U0LJcZQBd5XWt2rqhrPZj3e9YA-LPVk#how-to-train-endomorphs

strength. If you read about fitness or listen to podcasts about it, you might hear the term "achieving hypertrophy." Your ability to lift *a lot* of weight (a measure of strength) is not the same as your ability to grow your muscles.

It turns out that as an ectomorph, I need to consume more calories — and a lot of protein (which is the case for everyone) — in order to build muscle. Consuming a lot of calories when you're also doing intermittent fasting is a pretty tricky balance.

3

Understanding I was an ectomorph explained why building muscle felt like such an uphill battle. My fast metabolism and lean frame weren't character flaws — they were biological realities that required specific approaches. The challenge wasn't just about eating more or lifting heavier; it was about working with my natural body type rather than fighting against it or being ashamed of it. This realization shifted something in my mindset: what I'd seen as physical inadequacy was actually just a different starting point. But this raised new questions about pride and progress — if my body naturally responded differently to training, how should I feel about my achievements? Was I proud of working with my body type, or still comparing myself to different body types entirely?

In chapter 9 I wrote about having expectations based on what we see from fitness influencers and how that may be unrealistic because we're starting from different places and have different lives and different circumstances. There is a broader concept of comparison in general that is not usually helpful but definitely something we all do.

When I was in college I took a philosophy course my freshman year that was called "Ethics and Value Theory." The professor was awesome. This was the first course I remember from college and the first time I was exposed to the concept of philosophy from an educational perspective. Each time there was a class the professor opened with a single question. The rest of that day's class was devoted to discussion of the day's question. I always found it to be incredibly intellectually stimulating. With the established caveat that I'm a nerd — proudly — it was one of the only courses I took that I would continue to think about long after I had left the lecture hall.

One of those days, the question he posed to us was: "Do your parents love you?" The answer seemed obvious. Yes, of course. Multiple students answered as much. The professor followed up: "How do you know?"

For each response, he had a counter response but one of the student answers and the corresponding response from the professor seemed relevant to what we're discussing in this chapter. A student mentioned — in response to how they knew their parents loved them — that when they were a kid, their parents bought them things, provided a nice house, and played outside with them. The professor responded by asking that student if they thought the parents did all that because of love or because they wanted the neighbors to *see* that they were doing all those things; that the parents wanted it to *look* like they loved their kids because optics are important to people.

I won't get into the philosophical part of this debate. I believe my parents love me *just because* just like I love my kids *just because*.

The thing that struck me about that — and why I think it's relevant here — is that it really speaks to comparison. A parent might do something so that other parents will see that they are doing it and perhaps think or feel that they should also be doing it or ask why they aren't. The first parent in this situation is either motivated to do something because they are comparing themselves to the neighbor or hoping that the neighbor might make the comparison.

When my daughters were younger — and to a lesser extent even now — I found myself fighting the urge to compare them to other parents' children. I would also feel bad when I would sense that someone else was trying to compare their kids to mine. Is your daughter walking yet? Did you do potty training yet? Comparison, for me, feels a bit like a first cousin of jealousy. Jealousy is similar to making decisions when you're angry: nothing good comes from it.

Whether it's seeing a fitness influencer and thinking you'll never get to their level or seeing an advertisement in a magazine and thinking that what it shows is better than what you have or hearing from your friends that their kids have done something yours haven't, you aren't helping yourself get to your own goals. The comparison isn't helpful on its own. Using what you see or hear as information that helps to determine your own goals seems fine. That is a subtle distinction and perhaps just a semantic one from comparison. Allowing yourself to be driven by the information around you seems fine. The problem for me is born from being motivated to be someone else or to have what that person has. It's just not being fair to yourself.

This realization about comparison versus information-gathering helped shift my perspective on pride. If I could look at others' achievements as information rather than comparison points, maybe I could view my own progress the same way — not measuring against some ideal, but gathering data about what works for my body, my goals, and my journey.

4

Understanding that comparison wasn't serving me opened the door to something more valuable: authentic pride in genuine progress. Not pride measured against others' achievements or some idealized endpoint, but pride in the work, the consistency, and the willingness to understand my own body's needs.

Healthy self-regard, I've learned, isn't about constant validation or comparison. It's about maintaining a realistic view of both achievements and challenges. When I look in the mirror now, I try to see evidence of effort rather than measuring against some ideal. This shift from comparison to acknowledgment changes how progress feels — it becomes less about reaching a destination and more about appreciating the journey.

Self-regard is essentially how you consider yourself; and how much respect you have for yourself. A healthy amount of self-regard is made up of a few key components. Being able to acknowledge both your own strengths and weaknesses is important. We aren't perfect (well, maybe you are — but I'm not). Giving yourself grace — showing yourself compassion —

in the same way you'd show other people is also important. We are often our worst critics and harder on ourselves than we are on the people around us. Being able to recognize your limitations *and* your capabilities and acknowledge that you could develop and improve both is also a contributor to healthy self-regard.

All of that sounds straightforward but in practice might not be. The grass is always greener on the other side of the fence (speaking of comparisons). So how do you actually approach healthy self-regard in a practical way? We've talked about some of these things already. Setting and achieving small, and progressively iterative, goals is something you can do — right now. Recognizing that your hard work — your effort — is an achievement in and of itself. Outputs can be just as important as outcomes. Another tool you can use is measurement proof: those infamous progress photos and metrics or journals. It's easy to get down on yourself and sometimes it helps to have a reminder of the hard work you're putting in. When you look at those progress photos and nod your head or mark that you feel better today than you did yesterday, these are signals that you're developing a good sense of internal validation rather than relying solely on external validation.

Here is an example from my own experience. I recently took a break from intermittent fasting. I wanted to see if I could put on five to 10 pounds of weight and ideally muscle. Given how hard it has been for me to put on weight given my time-restricted eating, and knowing I could always go back to that, and also knowing that aside from intermittent fasting I've greatly improved my diet by eating better food and not eating the worse food, I figured it was a good opportunity to do a science experiment. Because of the intermittent fasting, I wasn't typically eating breakfast. So I decided to try and follow a nutrition plan and eat a protein-packed breakfast first thing in the morning. At the time I'm writing this paragraph, I have been eating the same breakfast for a week and a half: three eggs scrambled with cottage cheese mixed in, one apple, and a high-protein yogurt cup. For those counting macros, that works out to be around 560 calories and close to 50 grams of protein. Relatively speaking, it's a *ton* of food for me in the morning. There are a few things to note: I haven't had eggs in 20 years. I never loved them but didn't hate them either. I just never sought them out. I'm also not a good cook so scrambled is very easy for me to do. I don't like cottage cheese on its own but scrambling it into the eggs hides the taste and makes the eggs fluffier. Is it working? Am I shredded yet and have I put on the weight after one and a half weeks? No, and no to the second part. Is it working though? Absolutely but not for the reason you might think. After the first day, I took a picture of my meal and showed my wife. I was so proud of what I had done. Scrambled eggs don't make me Bobby Flay but for me, it may as well have. I also felt great because I tried something new that I know is healthy for me; I put in a new effort. Even if that effort hasn't yielded any noticeable results yet (and why would it) I still feel like I'm achieving something.

That was a shift for me. Before I would have gotten impatient that I didn't see results yet. I would have thought, "Anyone can scramble eggs" or "You're a grown-up Matt — eating cottage cheese isn't such a feat of greatness." Those would have ultimately been useless comparisons. This is my game. The act of doing it is now more important to me.

There are also warning signs that you might be skewing more towards an unhealthy self-regard. If you feel like a failure if you miss a workout or when you have a "cheat meal" it might be a good indicator that your self-regard isn't where it should be. We all have off days and we all enjoy a piece of chocolate cake (or the whole cake) from time to time. Enjoy it. It's ok. You aren't a failure. Acknowledging that you have made progress but feel like it's not enough — versus feeling like it's motivating you to want more — is another sign. If you catch yourself eating better or working out more because you are dependent on someone else's approval; not a good sign. If you just can't acknowledge that you've achieved anything you should try again.

Recognizing these warning signs helped me understand something crucial: the line between pride and vanity, between self-regard and self-absorption, isn't drawn by others — it's drawn by our relationship with our own progress.

Finding that line between healthy pride, shame, and vanity isn't about what others think — it's about developing an honest relationship with progress. Pride in achievement doesn't mean obsession with appearance. Being pleased with results doesn't mean becoming self-absorbed.

The goal isn't to eliminate pride — it's to understand it. To recognize that being proud of progress isn't vanity; it's acknowledgment of effort, commitment, and growth.

***

Something to think about...

What's the difference between pride and

vanity for you?

CHAPTER TWELVE

BEYOND AESTHETICS

1

Personal transformation has a ripple effect. What starts as individual change inevitably touches those around us — sometimes in ways we never expected. As my relationship with health and fitness evolved, I found myself navigating new territory: how to model healthy behaviors for my teenage daughters without projecting my own journey onto them, how to share achievements without making others feel diminished, how to balance being proud of progress while staying sensitive to others' paths.

The challenge wasn't just about achieving goals anymore — it was about understanding how those achievements affected my relationships, particularly as a father. When you're responsible for helping shape young minds, every action and every word about health and body image carries extra weight.

THE PARADOX OF FINE

We are all on our own journeys. Some of us might know or acknowledge it while others might not. I wonder if there's a single person anyone on Earth who, given truth serum, a mirror, and full transparency into their health, would honestly tell you that they believe they are perfectly fine just the way they are. I think we all can and do find flaws in ourselves or at the very least, things we'd like to improve. Count me among the group of people on Earth in this category. In addition, I imagine a series of concentric circles with me at the center. Within each circle is a different group of people in my life. The people in the inner-most circle are the people closest to me — my family. In the next circle out: my closest friends. As the circles get bigger and bigger, there are more and more people with progressively less and less of a relationship or even direct connection with me. Each person has this set of circles around them.

Each of the things that I do in life has some sort of effect on the people in my circles. Oftentimes, the people in the smallest circle — those closest to me — are the ones most affected by any actions I take. There are people in a circle so big and so far from the center that the actions I take have no impact on them. Each action is a stone being dropped right in the center, where I am. Each action is a different-sized stone. If I am going to the Red Sox game one night — a relatively small stone — that would mean I can't drive my daughters to a place they want to go. My attendance at that game would not only have no impact on, let's say, a co-worker, they might not even know I'm going.

If I were to run for, and become, the president of the United States that would have a massive impact on the inner circle and a meaningful impact on all my co-workers; even if it wasn't directly. Once elected, I would no longer be working at the company and that would affect them. In this case, the circles that are affected by my actions include the largest and most distant from the center.

At the beginning of my journey, as in before I was actually aware I needed to make any changes, my *lack* of action (to be or get healthy) had little to no impact on any of my circles but had it continued, certainly would have had a big impact on a number of them, most notably the inner-most circle where my family resides. I wouldn't have been around for very long and I'd like to think that my family would not have been thrilled with this as an outcome.

When I started to take action, the size of the metaphorical stone was small. Choosing to not drink soda doesn't mean someone else can't. I didn't ban soda from the house. I chose to exercise during times that wouldn't interfere with dad duties. As I progressed, the size of that stone got bigger. The potential for impact or to affect those closest to me also got bigger and so I had to start to be cognizant of those ripples; particularly for how they would affect my daughters and wife.

As the stone of my health journey grew larger, its ripples became more significant — particularly for my teenage daughters. Navigating these waters requires a delicate balance between modeling healthy behaviors and avoiding unintended consequences.

2

At the time when I started making changes to improve my health, my daughters were 12 and 13. These are formative years to be a teenage girl.

Here are some quotes from The National Organization for Women (NOW)[22]:

> "One study reports that At age thirteen, 53% of American girls are "unhappy with their bodies." This grows to 78% by the time girls reach seventeen."
>
> "45.5% of teens report considering cosmetic surgery"
>
> "40-60% of elementary school girls are concerned about their weight or about becoming 'too fat'."
>
> "46% of 9-11 year-olds are 'sometimes' or 'very often' on diets, and 82% of their families are 'sometimes' or 'very often' on diets.
>
> "Studies at Stanford University and the University of Massachusetts found that 70% of college women say they feel worse about their own looks after reading women's magazines."

These are not surprising pieces of information and as a father of teenaged daughters, something I'm always mindful of. I'm generally careful about what I talk about and what my daughters see me do. That was the case before I started getting healthier and needed to be the case during my health journey. All of a sudden I wasn't drinking soda and I wasn't eating breakfast and I wasn't eating as much junk anymore and I was exercising regularly. Over time — as my body started changing —

---

[22] NOW Body Image facts: https://now.org/now-foundation/love-your-body/love-your-body-whats-it-all-about/get-the-facts/

something my daughters may not have immediately noticed, my clothes changed too because things didn't fit me properly anymore. This was something they could notice.

The good news, I suppose, for my immediate family is that my wife and I established very early on that communication about anything and everything was on the table. We talk to them about anything they want to discuss — big, small, awkward, funny, sad, thoughtful, and all the things in between. The hope was (and has been proven to have worked for us) that they would feel comfortable talking to us anytime they had questions or concerns or things they were proud of and wanted to share. Just now, as I was typing the previous paragraph, my younger daughter sent me a text message with a screenshot of the results of her chapter 3 assessment test for her Algebra II class. She got an A+.

We also talk to them about trying alcohol, what "gummies" are — and not the fruit snack version, relationships, college prep, challenging situations with friends, and whatever else is on their minds. I figured I had to inform them about what I was doing — and why.

One night at the dinner table, I explained to them what was about to be going on in my life. I told them what little I knew about cholesterol at the time and how I wanted to be around and healthy for as long as possible. I wanted to meet my grandkids someday. This may have been a bit dramatic but was also true and my wife and I were nothing if not honest with our daughters. I told them this was about having a healthy heart.

I knew there could — and likely would — be other changes. I knew that my body might change and didn't want my daughters to see my dietary changes, my routine changes, and any potential physical changes to my body and think that I was doing any of these things for aesthetic reasons. I made sure to explain to them that I did not think I needed to lose any weight and that I was not unhappy with my body while at the same time acknowledging that a side effect of making healthier choices can be changes to your physical appearance. I've even gone so far as to invite them to exercise with me whenever they want. So far — now more than three years into this for me — I've had exactly zero takers.

For the most part, they seemed to understand my motivation and have never seemed to be bothered or negatively influenced (as far as I can tell) by the food and lifestyle changes I've made.

This understanding would sometimes manifest in unexpected ways. In the summer of 2023, I was in our pool chatting with some neighborhood parents we are friends with when my older daughter came out to say hello. I was standing in the shallow end which is just below waist deep for me. She crouched down by the pool's edge and whispered, surprisingly, "Dad! you have abs!" I found it funny — this was already two years into my journey, and she'd seen me in the pool many times. But that's often how changes register with kids — in random moments, without drama. I think she was proud of me. It was a pseudo-classic parent moment and frankly not surprising that my daughter basically never noticed this about me; even though we spend a lot of time together. It was as if she was saying, "Good work Dad."

Then there was one night, in February of 2024, when I got nervous.

I was out of the house for a meeting. My younger daughter sent me a text message and asked me if I could arrange for her to have a few sessions with the personal trainer I worked with. I replied and asked her pointedly — but trying not to lead — why? What were her goals? I knew at this point, more than two years into my new way of life, she had noticed how important exercise was to me, how important eating better had become for me, and that there had been some physical changes. I immediately feared that she was going to say that she wanted to improve something aesthetic. There was no particular reason for that fear — or anything she had done or said — other than my own sensitivity.

I wasn't sure how I would handle it if she said, "I want visible abs." As I watched the animated three-dot typing bubble on my screen the fear grew inside my head and in the pit of my stomach. I was really hoping that she had a good — a right — answer.

Finally, her message came in: "Can I say what I want on my body?"

Ugh.

"I would really like to get my arms stronger and maybe grow some muscle and I'd like to have more core and upper leg strength and stronger quads. I have a lot of strength in my calves already. I just want to be stronger."

A sigh of relief. Even if she actually and ultimately was interested in something aesthetic, she answered — in my mind — correctly.

She then sent another message: "I've told myself for a rly [really] long time that I wanted my body to be stronger but I never did anything abt [about] it and I know results take time but I want results to be before camp so I can continue on fitness."

I responded and asked if she would be willing to work, like really work, consistently. She told me she was. She then moved on to tell me how she wanted a digital camera. I was satisfied with her answers and arranged for her to have a few training sessions with the same trainer who I worked with. While the conversation may not have registered with her as any sort of big deal, for me it was validation that I had done a sufficient job of communicating why I was doing what I was doing and that any time anyone else wanted to try to get stronger or be healthier they were welcome to join.

Speaking of joining, my older daughter has no interest. I am writing this paragraph in December of 2024 a day after the following happened: this daughter has her driver's license and we've gotten used to her coming and going on her own. She came into the room where I was sitting and told me she was going to go to a local gym to exercise with one of her friends. I told her that she should just invite the friend over to use our home gym. She's more interested in going out to this particular gym with this particular friend. I say ok. About an hour later she came home, bouncing into that same room as if she were Winnie The Pooh's friend Tigger. She proceeded to tell me how much fun they had and asked if she could get a gym membership. She even tells me that she'll pay the monthly fee because she has a job now. I ask her why she wants to do that when we have all the equipment she needs in the basement.

"Dad. You don't even understand." She tells me that they have a Stair Master (which we don't have — although we do have regular stairs) but that she couldn't use it because it was occupied. She tells me that she walked on the treadmill and did some stretching and used the machine where your "legs go in and out" (hip abduction machine) and an assisted chin-up machine and a machine for abs that you put your knees on and rock back and forth. She was glowing (and not just from sweat). I asked her why she wanted to get the gym membership.

She explained that she had not just the friend who went that day but also a few other friends who liked going. She liked being in an environment where people were exercising and music was playing. She liked the experience of exercising with her friends. I told her that was all great and asked what her goal was. She told me she wanted to feel like she could run a mile and not be out of breath. She told me was happy with her weight but thinks it would be fun to have visible abs. I talked with her about how she should have a plan — that going to the gym was not a playground. If she actually wanted to achieve her goals she'd have to work really hard and be consistent and all the things she was talking about would need work outside of the gym too. She'd have to go to sleep earlier and maybe eat less junk food. She is a great communicator and tells us everything going on in her world so I felt pretty comfortable talking with her about all of this. During the entire conversation, she continued to bounce around in excitement of a new activity she wanted to try.

Today, the day after, she came home from work, ate a little dinner, got herself dressed in workout clothes, and went to the gym. She's excited to give it a go and I support the ambition. I even went as far as building her a little workout plan to try.

While navigating fitness discussions with my daughters required a particular sensitivity, I was also discovering that my transformation affected other relationships in different ways.

3

The conversation with my daughter about training highlighted something crucial: the difference between modeling behavior and prescribing it. While she had observed my journey for over two years, she came to her own conclusions about strength and fitness in her own time, for her own reasons. This was the balance I needed to find with everyone in my life — how to be authentic, realistic, and even proud about my journey while allowing others to not only find their own paths but to support them in ways that actually work for them and not in ways that *I think* would actually work for them.

I'm not a fitness influencer. I have never intended to be and I don't think I ever will be. I'm a software engineer. That's what I get paid to do. I'm not an expert on health or fitness or on any other person and not even an expert on myself; although at this point I'm pretty familiar with who and what I am. To think that anything I've done would exactly translate to anything you'd do is a fool's errand.

While I can't and shouldn't prescribe solutions for others, I can share what I've learned along the way. The key is understanding the difference between "here's what worked for me" and "here's what you should do." Just as my daughter found her own reason to pursue strength, everyone has their own motivation, timeline, and definition of success. Supporting others means accepting that their path might look nothing like mine.

I have had numerous conversations with a variety of friends over the handful of years since my journey started. Many of the conversations have a common theme: where do I start? What worked for you? Most of the people in this particular circle of friends have other things in common: we're all parents and all have jobs and generally busy lives. Most of us also share a "I used to be in good shape when I was younger" type of thing. Even if the goals someone else sets are the same as mine, the way they get there is likely to be very different. I have a different body type, different genetics, different metabolism, different medical history, different time constraints, different food tastes, and different things I enjoy. During these conversations, I am always willing to talk about the various things I've tried and share what's worked for me but am certainly mindful that it is all based on my own experience. I make it a point to explain that while I tried intermittent fasting, cutting out soda, starting to track macronutrients, exercising regularly, and so on, I don't really know how to articulate what the individual contributions of each of those things were. I explain that in a real science experiment, it would be better to try one thing at a time and measure its impact. This is how we introduce solid foods to babies — one at a time — to make sure there aren't any allergies or digestion issues. In my case, I figured it would be easier to do whatever the opposite of cold turkey is and just start everything all at once.

The plan worked well for me because I'm the type of person who thrives on routines and I'm generally really organized. Because of my engineering background, I also deal with a good number of obsessive-compulsive tendencies. In this particular case, that is a big advantage. That just might not work for other people.

When my wife and I were interviewing pediatricians before our first daughter was born, the doctor we ultimately picked was someone who was willing to tell us what she would do if it were her child. Other pediatricians we met with were a bit more wishy-washy and less direct. This isn't to say that we have to agree or have to follow the advice that we're given exactly. That's not what it's about. We wanted someone to give us information that was at least somewhat influenced by their own experience who would trust us to use that information to make the decisions that worked for our family; for us.

I want the autonomy to make decisions about what's right for me and not feel like I'm being forced or pressured into doing something because someone else is *positive* that it is the right solution for everyone. If that information has come from a friend and something about what they had prescribed didn't seem right to me, I'm certain it would make me feel like I was letting them down. At that point, my goals have become about *them* instead of being about *me*.

I don't want to feel like I'm letting someone down. I want to feel like I'm being supported; like I'm being encouraged. This is why the fitness influencer realm is so dangerous: if you want to look like this (the influencer) then you just have to do what I do.

This feels like a form of the transitive property to me: if it were that simple, we'd all be shredded. We aren't all shredded so therefore, it's not that simple. It's not simple because you and I aren't that person. We're us.

When people ask me for information or help I try very hard to share what I can but without any judgment and with as much understanding as possible. I'm proud of what I've achieved so far but also acknowledge that it's specific to me. In the same way that I've learned from the achievements of others, particularly people with relatable experiences, I try to never preach.

Understanding how to balance personal achievement with sensitivity to others' journeys isn't just about being considerate — it's about creating sustainable change that positively affects everyone in our circles. As I moved forward, this balance would become crucial for maintaining progress — not just in physical health, but in the relationships that support lasting change.

***

Something to think about...

How might your health journey affect those around you?

PART FIVE

THE LONG VIEW

CHAPTER THIRTEEN

BETTER THAN FINE

1

"Fine" had been my comfort zone for decades. It was safe, acceptable, and undemanding. But once I was given so much evidence that it required me to stop accepting "fine" in my health, I also started questioning "fine" in other areas of my life. Like a loose thread that, when pulled, starts to unravel the whole sweater, challenging "fine" in one area of life inevitably leads to examining it in others.

Dr. Carol Dweck, a psychologist, talks about the concepts of a fixed mindset versus a growth mindset[23]. The former is how much someone believes that their basic qualities — like intelligence and talent — are fixed or permanent. The latter is when someone believes those same qualities can be changed or evolved. It's possible that in certain areas of your life, you have a

---

[23] Mindset Works: https://www.mindsetworks.com/science/

fixed mindset and a growth mindset in other areas. Generally speaking, when you believe you can improve in some way and are willing to do the work in order to do so, you are more likely to achieve more; to grow.

This concept of fixed versus growth mindset plays out differently across different aspects of our lives. Someone might have a growth mindset about their career but a fixed mindset about their physical capabilities. Or vice versa. Recognizing where we hold fixed mindsets is often the first step to challenging them.

When you hear yourself saying or even just thinking, "You can't teach an old dog new tricks," you're succumbing to a fixed mindset. This is much more likely the older you get. Maybe it's because you don't think you can do something better than you've done before. Maybe you think you can't learn something new. Maybe you just don't feel like you have the energy or time.

I think there's an added challenge. There was never an acute moment for me when I could identify that I was now getting older and would no longer be putting effort into my health. For most people, it isn't a binary switch where one day you just stop caring or stop trying. In the past couple of years, I've had two coworkers suffer pretty serious injuries — tearing an ACL and tearing an Achilles tendon. Both of them happened while participating in sports activities that they'd both done many times before. In our office, when they both returned to action, these were the moments when they realized they weren't as young as they used to be; that maybe they can't do the same things they used to do in the same ways they used to do them. While I don't wish for anyone to hurt themselves or be injured in any way, those moments often act as "wake-up calls" and can cause someone to stop an activity entirely rather than figure out how to evolve their participation.

These moments of realization — whether through injury, blood work, or other wake-up calls — present a choice: retreat to what feels safe or adapt how we engage with challenges. The comfort zone isn't just physical — it's psychological. And understanding how to push its boundaries without breaking ourselves becomes crucial for continued growth.

2

Fine feels safe. Fine is comfortable. It doesn't make a ton of logical sense to ever want to be uncomfortable. Our comfort zone is the place where we feel safe with the least amount of stress. It is very challenging to intentionally choose to leave that zone and it gets harder and harder the older you get. The comfort zone encourages the sense of being "fine" and being "fine" is the equivalent of settling to stay in your current comfort zone.

The first step to whatever is better than fine, for you, is to accept that you will likely have to step outside of your existing comfort zone. I don't drink coffee and I don't drink alcohol. Drinking soda felt like my biggest vice and a drink that made me feel comfortable. It was my go-to beverage. It was what I ordered at every restaurant and the movie theater and while I was watching TV at home. It was what I drank with every meal other than breakfast. I definitely had a moment where I considered if I could get away with simply cutting back the volume of soda.

Maybe I could stay in my soda comfort zone but just shrink it a bit. Ultimately I decided that there was less risk for me to cut it out entirely. If I had told myself that I was "allowed" one soda a day or three sodas a week or whatever the rule would be, it would be very simple to see a situation where those three sodas a week turned into five sodas a week. One a day could easily turn into one most days but some days I'd have two. It made me comfortable to drink soda and the idea of not drinking soda at all was an uncomfortable thought.

But I did it. I cut out soda entirely and it didn't take long for my mind to reassure me that I'd be fine. People do hard things all the time. Deciding to not drink soda anymore probably doesn't make it to the Mount Rushmore of difficult challenges people have accomplished but for me, it was a big deal.

What's interesting about comfort zones is how they shrink or expand based on our choices. Each time we stay within them, they tend to contract, making future changes feel even more daunting. But when we push their boundaries, even slightly, they begin to expand, making the next challenge feel more manageable. It's like giving yourself room to breathe.

I was nervous before my first workout with my personal trainer. I was nervous going to that hot Pilates class I mentioned back in chapter 5. I was incredibly nervous about taking that first progress photo. I was nervous about modifying my diet and about what I would eat instead of going to McDonald's for a double quarter pounder at least a few times a week. For each of these things, I had to step outside of my own personal comfort zone to try something new to me in the service of doing something better for me. Each time I did it there was a little more evidence that made the next time the slightest bit easier.

I don't mean to minimize or oversimplify how hard it is to step out of your comfort zone but ultimately it is something you need to do if you are going to grow. Research shows that operating slightly outside our comfort zone — in what psychologists call the 'optimal anxiety' zone — actually improves performance and accelerates personal growth. Too much comfort can be as detrimental to progress as too much stress.

There's a psychological concept called the Yerkes-Dodson law[24]. It basically says that someone reaches their peak level of performance with an intermediate level of stress. In other words, just getting a bit out of your comfort zone, which is stressful and anxiety-inducing, is ultimately the way to promote higher performance. It is literally the way you build muscle. In order for your muscles to grow you actually have to stress them to the point of causing small tears. These tears then heal stronger and cause your muscles to grow bigger than before.

The Yerkes-Dodson law can be represented by an upside-down 'U'. Start by picturing an upside-down 'U' on a chart where the X axis is stress level and the Y axis is performance. The bottom left would be low stress and low performance (your comfort zone). The bottom right would be high stress and low performance (pushing yourself too hard which is ultimately not productive and could be detrimental to your health). The sweet spot is in the middle of the X-axis and the top of the Y-axis. Here

---

[24] Healthline - What the Yerkes-Dodson Law Says About Stress and Performance: https://www.healthline.com/health/yerkes-dodson-law

you are experiencing some — but not too much — stress and optimal performance. That's what we're aiming for.

YERKES-DODSON LAW BELL CURVE

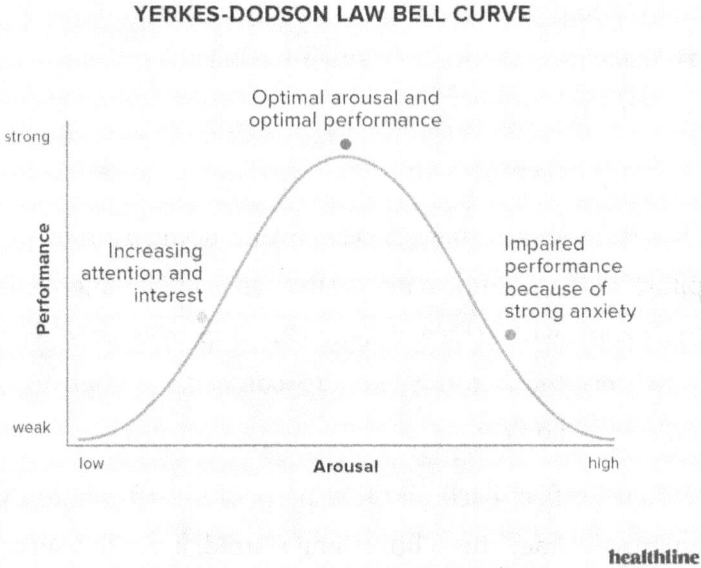

This principle appears everywhere in life, not just in physical training. Learning new skills, tackling creative projects, and even building relationships — all require finding that stress sweet spot between comfort and overwhelming challenge. Too little stress leads to stagnation; too much leads to burnout.

Understanding this sweet spot between comfort and excessive stress changed how I approached challenges. Just as I learned to find the right amount of stress in exercise — enough to grow but not so much to injure — I started seeing opportunities for productive discomfort in other areas of my life. The evidence was clear: growth happens at the edge of comfort, not in its center.

3

The fascinating thing about pushing comfort zones is how the benefits compound. Each small victory builds confidence for the next challenge, creating a positive feedback loop of growth and achievement.

Growth begets growth.

Research shows that success in one domain often creates a "spillover effect," improving performance in seemingly unrelated areas. People who achieved significant improvements in one area of life were much more likely to succeed in other areas than people who didn't.

When I reflect back on other parts of my life where I've also seen growth since this whole thing started, it doesn't seem like it is a coincidence. The growth associated with figuring out my health and fitness gave me a lot more confidence in my personal life. This confidence translated to other areas and aspects of my life.

I spent almost a decade trying to figure out how and what to write my first book about. There were many false starts before it all clicked and I felt like I actually figured out what to write about and how to write it. The idea of writing a book was daunting. I had been asking myself where to even start. Who would care about anything I write? Why would they care? I finally had the confidence or at the very least less of a concern about what other people would think. This creative confidence or reduced inhibition grew alongside the physical confidence.

Also, as I've referenced earlier in the book, I grew up being known and called "the skinny kid." Skinny — for guys — is generally considered to be undesirable. I've definitely heard women tell each other — or even me in my adult life — "I wish I was as skinny as you are." I have never been told that by another guy at any stage of my life. This isn't me passing judgment on the concept of "skinny" but in guy-hood, wrongly, by the way, being skinny is often associated with being weak. I never felt strong in the conventional sense. I always felt quite a bit of confidence in my intellect and while I was a good athlete, overpowering people on the basketball court, baseball diamond, or tennis courts was not my modus operandi. I am also a decent chess player. The skills to be good at chess are more like the skills that I used to make me good at sports.

Strength, however, means something different for me now. Strength is more than just how far you can hit the baseball, how fast your serve is, or if you can run through a screen that the defender sets. It's not even about how much weight you can bench. Strength is about accepting that I haven't done things exactly right. It's about how willing I am to ask for help. It's accepting that I don't need to be the best at something or even know how to do it at all to give it a try. Strength is being willing to fail. Strength is caring less about what other people think and more about how you feel. Strength is feeling proud of your effort.

Strength is discovering a new confidence in a part of your life where it previously didn't exist.

This new understanding of strength — as something that encompasses both physical and mental resilience — changed how I viewed progress itself. It wasn't just about getting stronger or healthier anymore; it was about building a sustainable approach to growth that could last beyond any single achievement. The question became: how do you maintain this momentum without burning out?

What started as a high cholesterol reading became a catalyst for questioning "fine" everywhere. Physical strength led to mental strength. Health goals sparked creative confidence. Each small step beyond comfort created momentum for the next one.

The evidence was clear: "fine" wasn't just a state of being — it was a choice. And once you choose to question it in one area, you start to see possibilities for growth everywhere. The challenge isn't finding opportunities to be better than fine — it's having the courage to take that first step beyond being comfortable.

***

Something to think about...

In what other areas of your life have you been accepting "fine?" What do you think lies beyond those comfort zones?

CHAPTER FOURTEEN

HEALTH SPAN

1

The ultimate paradox of transformation isn't about how we change — it's about how we maintain that change. After questioning "fine," pushing comfort zones, and discovering hidden strengths, the real challenge becomes sustainability: how do we turn these changes into a lifestyle that lasts?

Acknowledging that you need to make changes is the first step and ultimately — while perhaps the hardest step — is also the step that requires the least amount of effort. It's what happens after you make that decision that takes the most effort and the most resolve. Without that effort and without the resolve to continue on you are not likely to reach your goals. This is why so many people go through lots of starts and stops; particularly at the beginning of each calendar year. The idea of change sounds great but the practice of change is much harder.

There are two types of change (well, three if you count the cash and coin situation when purchasing things without a credit card or Venmo): change and lasting change. Starting something is the change. Deciding to go on a diet, deciding to start a workout program, and choosing to look for a new job are all examples of potential change. Lasting change is when the effort associated with the change becomes natural and automatic; a routine that you follow. Once you've developed sustainable eating habits or when you start loving exercise as part of your daily life or when you start sending your resume out are all examples of lasting change.

Change has an endpoint and is about outcomes: I'm going to improve my triglycerides. Lasting change is ongoing and emphasizes the process: health and fitness are part of my daily routine to the point where I don't even think about triglycerides anymore. Change is thinking about commitment and lasting change is about demonstrating it.

But how do we make this transition from the initial change to lasting change? The answer might lie in how we view our goals themselves. When we focus solely on the endpoint — that final number on the scale, that target cholesterol reading, that ideal physique — we often miss something crucial: the path to get there. It's like standing at the base of a mountain, eyes fixed only on the distant peak and imaging what's on the other side, missing all the crucial footholds that will actually get us there.

2

I'm not a good artist so I won't try to illustrate an example of the mountain. I will, however, try to describe it in a way that connects back to the original motivation for me to improve my own health.

Picture me standing at the base of that mountain. It's a giant mountain. I can't see what's on the other side of it but I know that my goal — the treasure — is waiting for me on the other side. I can see the top of the snow-capped mountain but there is tall grass, trees, and boulders between me and that top. I can't actually see the path I need to take but I know — at least I think I know — where I need to go. I just want to get there as fast as possible and my gut tells me I should go up that mountain. As I stand at the base of the mountain, sure of where I need to get but unsure of how to get there, it can be quite daunting. I start walking and before I know it, I have reached an obstacle I didn't see coming: a river that runs through the path I was following with no apparent way around. It's too deep to walk across and the current is strong and bonus: I am not a good swimmer. I'm stuck. I decide it's not worth continuing because if it's already this challenging and already taking this long, I'll never get to the treasure.

Even if I make it across the river, what I didn't know was that there are more obstacles; some trickier to navigate than others. There is a pack of bears, maybe a chasm with a rickety rope bridge I can use to cross with planks that randomly fall out, or a random pool of lava! Who knows? The journey becomes exhausting and is filled with opportunities to turn around and give up. So that's what I did.

Now let's look at it with a different approach for my second attempt. The big goal — getting to that treasure — is still the same but this time, I'm not looking beyond the first steps; beyond the first obstacle. This time, I know the river is coming so I'm prepared. All I'm concerned with at the moment is getting across that river. When I get to the river's edge, I look around and figure out that there's a shallow and narrow area that I can walk across safely. I have achieved my first small goal. It isn't until right now that I start thinking about the next small goal: the pack of bears. I now think of what my strategy will be for circumventing the bears. I take a really long detour but make it around the bears before I reach the chasm.

I won't bore you with all the details for each of the obstacles but this attempt, with its set of small goals that all iteratively help me reach the large goal, feels much more approachable. In its totality, it still requires the same if not more effort and is probably just as daunting but because I'm approaching each obstacle deliberately it's easier to think through the right solution for me; one step at a time. This also gives me the opportunity to pivot — or circumvent — along the way as necessary. There are fewer surprises.

The idea of eating an entire pizza feels ridiculous to me. The idea of eating a slice of pizza — six times — feels much more possible.

This iterative approach to goals doesn't just make them more achievable — it makes the changes more sustainable. When we break down overwhelming transformations into manageable steps, we build confidence and competence along the way. Each small victory becomes a foundation for lasting change.

3

So how do we actually break down these seemingly insurmountable goals into achievable pieces? The answer lies in working backward — starting with the end goal and identifying the stepping stones that will get us there. In my case, "lower cholesterol" wasn't specific enough. I needed concrete, measurable steps. In retrospect, what I should have done was eliminate soda this week, learn about nutrition next week, and start basic exercise the week after. Each piece needed to be both challenging enough to matter and small enough to achieve. What I actually did was all of those things at the same time and while it ultimately worked for me, in hindsight with what I know now, that was a risky approach and I'm lucky it didn't fail.

The key is making each goal specific and achievable while understanding that the path might shift as we learn. Just as I discovered different obstacles on my mountain journey, we often uncover new challenges — and new opportunities — as we progress.

In this book, I've talked about goal setting, progress tracking, and celebrating achievements. They are all connected. By setting those small goals you are making it easier to track your progress and giving yourself more opportunities to celebrate your achievements.

Let's look more closely at a version of the plan I probably should have followed:

Step 1: Track my current eating habits. While I was certainly familiar with the food and drink I was consuming, I wasn't tracking it. I had no real idea about how much or what kinds of food or soda I was eating and drinking. Tracking, even for a short period of time, would have given me a baseline.

Step 2: Eliminate soda. If I had done this as a discreet action rather than as part of the bundle, I would have been able to compare it to the previously set baseline and know what its actual effect was.

Step 3: Learn about macronutrients. From step 1 I would have had a baseline understanding of what I was eating and now I'd learn what was in all those foods, what was good for me, what wasn't good for me, and how much of each macro I needed.

Step 4: Start walking 15 minutes per day. This would have been the least risky way to start exercising in a deliberate way. I would not have needed to stay at this level for very long — probably only a few days — before this habit would have been formed.

Step 5: Make healthier food choices. This is where I'd start to consume more protein and less saturated fat. This is also where I'd be mindful of the time of day I was eating (like not eating too late at night) even if I wasn't going to start doing intermittent fasting.

Step 6: Add strength training. Now that I had a better understanding of my nutrition, had cut out some of the negative food influences, and started the habit of walking, it would be time to start building muscle. This is probably where I'd start working with a personal trainer — or at the very least follow a program designed by a professional.

These steps are all things that I essentially merged into one big step but splitting them up into separate parts would have been easier to measure. Each time I took one of those steps I'd have a reason to celebrate in some small way. Each celebration would build momentum and make the next step just a little bit easier and a lot more enticing.

This step-by-step approach doesn't just make goals more achievable — it makes success more measurable and sustainable. Each small victory builds not just confidence, but understanding. As these individual changes become habits, they create a foundation for lasting transformation. The question then becomes: how do we maintain this momentum for the long run?

4

When I started this journey, I was focused on numbers: cholesterol readings and triglycerides followed eventually by body fat percentage. But somewhere along the way, the goal shifted from fixing specific problems to building a better future. This wasn't just about living longer — it was about living better. The concept of "health span" — the quality of our years, not just the quantity — became increasingly important.

For my life, I hope to have a high quantity of high-quality years. I want both. There's the old cliche about how getting old sucks, but it doesn't have to. Perhaps it is too reductive to just say that you have a choice. There are so many things that are outside of our control. The reality is that despite my best efforts, some unforeseen event could happen that would cost me my health or worse, my life. I can't worry about the things I can't control. I frankly don't want to worry about the things I can control. I'd rather just do something about it.

I know it sounds easy and I know it actually isn't. I know it sounds, as my daughters would call it, cringy. I looked up the definition of the word *lucky*. The first definition in the dictionary[25] is "having good luck." The second definition is "happening by chance" followed by "producing or resulting in good by chance." I don't know if those are helpful definitions but I *feel* like I got lucky with my journey and its success so far; but not by chance. I went to an annual and routine doctor's appointment and found out my cholesterol was at dangerously high levels. This wasn't chance. It was the result of a buildup of bad habits over decades. These habits seemed innocuous on their own. Had they not, I probably would have made changes much earlier.

I seemed ok but clearly wasn't. It didn't happen overnight. For many people, there are warning signs. I might have been just as likely or just as at risk to have a heart attack as someone who was obese. I looked relatively healthy so I must have been, right? Wrong.

The paradox of fine is that when you perceive yourself as being fine you are less likely to look for opportunities to grow let alone actually strive to do so. By not putting in that work, you

---

[25] Merriam-Webster Dictionary: https://www.merriam-webster.com/dictionary/lucky

will inevitably be less fine; particularly as you age. Being fine implies being settled. Being settled implies not wanting to change. Not changing leads to stagnation and degradation with age.

I felt fine and then realized the hard way that it wasn't enough. Maybe it seems obvious but I had to look closely at the way I was living my life — at the details — in order to see and learn what was really going on. What I ended up seeing was surprising and in many cases, not pretty but because I looked closely, I could ultimately see what I needed to see in order to catalyze change.

In July of 2024, I had my annual checkup with Kaitie again. The focus is no longer on triglycerides. I've got that under control. This time, she asked me if I wanted them to test something called Lipoprotein (a). She explained that high levels of Lipoprotein (a) are an indicator of a higher risk of heart attack or stroke down the line. It is mostly inherited (genetic) and can affect anyone, regardless of other health factors. I asked her why I *wouldn't* want to test that. She explained that some people just don't want to know since it's genetic and there would be limited recourse. While there are new medications and treatments, they aren't well-developed yet. I didn't hesitate. Yes, I want to know. If there was an underlying problem — even if it was genetic — I wanted to know so I could do whatever I needed to mitigate as much risk as possible.

Prior to July of 2021, I don't think I would have answered yes to her question. It would have been scary for me. I would have been afraid. My perception of fine would be better served by not looking too closely at anything and not disrupting my status quo.

This is perhaps the ultimate paradox of "fine" — that accepting "fine" actually prevents us from being truly fine. When we hide behind "fine," we miss opportunities not just for improvement, but for discovery. What started as a mission to fix one health marker became a journey that revealed how much lay hidden beyond "fine." The real treasure wasn't just in better health numbers or stronger muscles — it was in finding the courage to look beyond comfortable acceptance.

So now, I'm not afraid of what I'll see if I look. I'm curious about what I'll miss if I don't.

ACKNOWLEDGMENTS

While I've dedicated this book to my family, there are many others whose support and guidance made both this journey and this book possible.

To Kaitie: I know you aren't *technically* a doctor. But you're still *my* doctor. So often — more often than not — a doctor would prescribe medication to someone who hit the cholesterol levels I hit but your faith in me and willingness to help me come up with a plan were the fundamental building blocks of confidence that I could actually do it. I fully believe that you saved my life.

To Liz: I was your first client and you were my first personal trainer on this journey. Thanks for showing me how to exercise the right way and helping me fall in love with the idea of taking better care of myself.

To my friends and family who have suffered through years of hearing me talk about my journey and who are inevitably reading this book out of a sense of obligation: your support is invaluable.

To you: thank you for taking the time to read this book. I hope you have found it to be interesting, maybe a little informative, and maybe a little funny.

Also, for everyone reading this: I hope you don't feel like I was judging you or ever making it seem like any of this is easy for me to say or easy for you to do. It's hard work and takes a lot of patience, discipline, and resolve — but I know you can do it.

Get to work.

www.ingramcontent.com/pod-product-compliance
Lightning Source LLC
Chambersburg PA
CBHW072138270326
41931CB00010B/1796